Dedication

*To our children: Cara and Julie; Debra, Jeff, and Barry
—for sharing the joy of play with us.
To our husbands: Ken and Sid
—for continued support in our endeavors.*

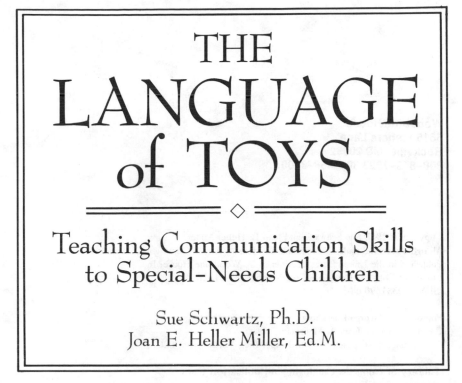

THE
LANGUAGE
of TOYS

◇

Teaching Communication Skills
to Special-Needs Children

Sue Schwartz, Ph.D.
Joan E. Heller Miller, Ed.M.

A Guide for Parents and Teachers

WOODBINE HOUSE • 1988

Woodbine House
5615 Fishers Lane
Rockville, MD 20852
800–843–7323/301–468–8800

Published in the United States of America by Woodbine House, Inc.
Library of Congress Catalogue Card Number: 87-51320
ISBN: 0-9331490-08-5

Photographs: George Rosenberg
Cover Illustration: Gary A. Mohrmann
Book Design & Typesetting: Wordscape, Inc., Washington, D.C.

Library of Congress Cataloging-in-Publication Data
Schwartz, Sue
    The language of toys.

    Bibliography: p.
    Includes index.
    1. Language acquisition. 2. Educational toys.
    3. Slow learning children–Language. I. Miller,
Joan E. Heller. II. Title.
P118,S293 1988   649'.15   87-51320
ISBN 0-933149-08-5 (pbk.)

Manufactured in the United States of America

    4 5 6 7 8 9 10

Acknowledgements

Our thanks to:

The staff at Woodbine House for their faith in our abilities to help children develop their language skills through play.

The parents and children who agreed to be photographed during their playtime.

Judy and Peter Black
Lois and Amanda Cheney
Joanne and Stephanie Corbin
Chris, Stevie, and Justin Dignan
Flo Ritter and Jimmy Etheridge
Aya Kitmitto
Patty and Lauren Mahaffey
Joan and Cara Miller
Jim Peters
Mike and Michael Seraphin
Irv and Jake Shapell
Putryrom, Christopher, and Vlady Vy
Pam and Thomas Williams

George Rosenberg for his patience and excellent photography.

Dr. Melvin Heller for his literary genius.

Amy, Hayley, and Nanci for their help in typing.

All of our friends and colleagues for their advice and encouragement for this work.

Table of Contents

Introduction

Developing communication is as much a basic human need as seeking food and comfort. For many children this is a relatively simple process, while for others there may be significant delays in this area. There are a wide variety of causes for a language delay in some children. Regardless of the cause, the results are usually the same: a child with delayed language development and concerned parents.

These concerned parents want to help their children with special needs learn language skills but often don't know the best way to go about it. Through our years of teaching and raising our own children, we have seen that an amazing amount of language can be pulled from even the simplest toy. Our book, *The Language Of Toys*, shows you how to use toys to aid your child's language development. While you are playing with your child, you can be helping him increase his language skills. And you can have fun together at the same time. We know your child can benefit from these times with Mom and Dad. We also know this play/work time is dramati-

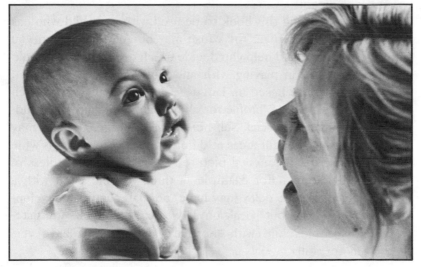

cally more important for children with delays in their language development. They will need the extra effort that their parents can give them to help develop their language skills.

When speech and language therapists or teachers work with children with language delays, they usually use toys they think will encourage certain words or sounds. There is no "magic" to the toys they use. Rather, the toys are chosen carefully to be teaching aids. This book will help you to choose and to use toys like the professionals to enhance the development of language in *your* child. Although we have selected certain toys for this book, we want to assure you that there are many other toys that can be bought or made which can serve equally well.

The Language Of Toys is divided into two parts. In the first part, we explain important background information about language, its sequential development, some of the causes of language delay, the value of play, how play can enhance language development, and your role in all this. In the next section—which is the heart of the book—we recommend toys that we have found to be useful in stimulating language development and show you how to use these toys in playing with your child. For each toy in the book we provide you with sample language dialogues to help you get the most from that toy. We encourage you to use these ideas in your play as well as to go beyond and devise new ways of playing to encourage language development.

We have designed this book to be used with any child who has a language delay, whatever the cause may be. We have given you guidelines which should help you decide which toys your child would be most interested in playing with and most ready to learn from. These guidelines are based on language developmental ages. Each child has his own unique profile for all developmental areas, including cognition, motor, social, self-help, *and* language. A child may make progress in different areas at different rates. The result is wide variation in the developmental picture for each child, regardless of his chronological age. For example, a three-year-old child with a twelve month language delay may have "normal" cognitive development or motor skills but speak on a two-year-old level. Alternately, a four-year-old child with "normal" language may have very delayed motor skills.

We have individual suggestions for modifying your play to accommodate the specific learning needs of each child. We are sure that we haven't addressed every individual need but we feel that you will be able to adapt our suggestions to your own child. The toys and exercises in this book are arranged by language developmental ages. Each section covers several months and presents toys and dialogues that are appropriate for your child's particular level of language development. There are similar guidelines throughout the book to help you pick toys that are the most appropriate for your child's level of language development.

In addition to toys you can buy, we also include at least two homemade toys for each of our language developmental levels. Many people enjoy making toys and there is a lot of benefit—including saving money—in this. In our work, we have found that children and parents treasure these homemade toys long after other toys have been packed away.

Remember, our suggestions are only suggestions. Expand and create. There are many books in libraries and in bookstores which will tell you more about homemade toys. We have included several in our reference list at the back of this book.

Parents often ask, "When should we start?" You can start the exercises in this book even before your child's language delay has been formally diagnosed. If you already know that your child has some special needs, you have to consider the possibility that he is language delayed too. Do not wait until you have a specific diagnosis of language delay to begin. Often your child's diagnosis has to wait until you are able to test him and in many cases that doesn't happen before age two. You can always work on his language skills even before getting a diagnosis. It can only help him in the long run. As you will see in our chapter on language development, you would not expect your child to be talking in understandable language much before one year of age. We want you to enrich your child's language long before that time.

If your child is an older preschooler and you have just gotten the diagnosis of a language delay, then you can start this book at whatever level your child is placed and work from there. You might even be working with a therapist or school at this time. Show them this book and explain how you want to integrate our ideas with your

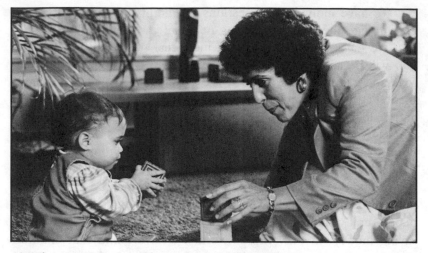

child's specific plan. You will probably find that our examples fit right in with your child's individual education plan.

We do not expect, or want, you to turn into a teacher for your child or to lose your role of parent. However, you can combine both roles in a way that is fun for both you and your child. There is also no need to occupy your child's every waking moment with the exercises in this book. There are times when children should play alone because that is when they build independence and develop imagination. We believe, however, that parents, teachers, families, babysitters, and others can enhance the development of richer language by playing with toys with children for *part* of the child's playtime.

Follow your child's lead. If he is interested in farm animals, explore that area in your play. If you see that he has no interest at all in cars and trucks, then put that idea aside for a while. Your play should be fun, interesting, and meaningful. Experience *your* childhood again and enjoy the time you will spend in playful learning with your child.

One

Language: An Introduction

Language is everywhere. It is everywhere we live and work; and it will be everywhere our children will live and work too. There is almost nothing we or our children do in this world that does not

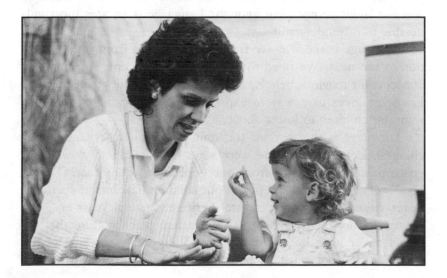

involve some type of communication. It is one of the most important life skills our children can acquire.

This chapter reviews some of the basics of language: what language is, its importance to society and how it develops.

The Need For Language In Our Society

Society could not function without language to explain complex inventions, convey ideas, or relay information. History, science, law, technology, and mathematics are all based on information. And that information can only be communicated through language. We use language to record our past, to chart our present, and to prepare for our future. Our children will need language in order to participate fully in all these activities of our society. They will need language to participate fully in their own personal worlds as well.

Language is the way we explain our feelings. How could we express our deepest emotions without language? Fear, anger, happiness, and sadness are all communicated using language. All through life people use language in forming relationships, expressing love, and sharing thoughts and feelings.

Language, with its many nuances, is more art than science. How often have we found ourselves trying to explain our way out of situations caused by faulty communication? "That is not what I meant; you misunderstood what I said." Did he or she misunderstand or was our language not clear enough? Language is an area most vulnerable to misunderstanding.

Language is the way we transmit our values from one generation to the next. We need to communicate concepts for morality, concepts for religious beliefs, and concepts for family expectations. Language gives us a way to express things we've never seen but want our children to know about.

Language is the way we transmit our cultural heritage to our children. Long before there were ways to write things down, language passed on legends from one generation to another. Telling vivid stories of people and places our children have never seen and never visited passes on a cultural heritage. Several years ago, the powerful story of *Roots* gave us insight into black culture that we would never have known otherwise. The graphic retelling of the events of the Holocaust keeps that part of our history alive. Each year at Christmas and Easter, the retelling of the story of Jesus fascinates a new generation.

Language is a vital tool for our special needs children to have, for it is through language—whether spoken, signed, pointed to, or combinations of all three—that they will reach their fullest potential. In order for us to help our children reach that potential, it is important that we understand how language develops. With that knowledge, we can decide how to best help our children.

Special needs children should be evaluated on an individual basis and have learning goals set specifically for them. When you learn how language develops, you can decide where on the continuum your child is now and begin working to strengthen her language skills from that point. Understanding the basics of language development is the first step.

Language Development

The development of language in young children is exciting. Parents everywhere share the excitement of that first coo or gurgle that actually sounds like "mama" or "dada." The long distance telephone companies profit from countless phone calls to Grandma and Grandpa who wait in breathless anticipation as the little one breathes into the phone for ten minutes and finally gurgles out that "first word." How do we get to that first word? Is the first coo or gurgle a "true" word? Did we teach our child that "first word" or did she develop language on her own?

This section will answer these and many more questions about the development of language. We are actually taught our native language by living with and interacting with people all around us. Many of us acquire language easily and without effort, while others will need special teaching to attain all the language that is possible.

One of the things we need to talk about is the difference between speech and language.

Receptive Language, Expressive Language, And Speech

The question Grandmas, Grandpas, and friends ask often is, "Is she talking yet?" What they are really asking is "Does she have *expressive language* yet?" We can't answer that question until we learn what receptive language, expressive language, and speech mean. We have to have receptive language before we can have anything more than the most basic expressive language. We need both receptive language and expressive language to have communication.

Receptive Language is the information that your child takes in. It is what she hears all around her. It is what she understands. For example, if a child is asked, "Where's the doggie?" she will look around and point to Rover. This will show that she *understands* what was asked even though she may not yet be able to say "Rover" or "doggie." Children must be exposed to receptive language in order to develop communication skills. The language they are exposed to early in life is crucial to developing these skills.

Fortunately most young children are surrounded daily by language which they hear from brothers, sisters, neighbors, TV, radio and YOU. Even when you don't think you're "teaching" your child language, you are. You are because you are talking and she is listening! Basic human communication can be as simple as this or can be enriched in ways we talk about later.

Before you can answer that question, "Is she talking yet?" with a proud "YES," your child must have receptive language–language that she hears around her and that she understands. After many hours and several months of listening, you'll be rewarded with that first precious word. Be sure to call everybody you know with the good news and tell them that she is "talking;" you'll know that what she is really doing is using expressive language.

Expressive Language begins with the birth cry. As air rushes across your infant's vocal cords, she announces her arrival in the world. You receive her message and understand, so you have your first communication with your newborn. Expressive language is the communication of one person to another. It can be through crying, through laughter, through words, through gestures, through a formal system of sign language or combinations of any of these. If we go back to our example of the child and the dog, we would expect that if the child has expressive language that she would be able to point to the dog and in some manner produce the word for "doggie" or "Rover." This is now *expressive* language.

Speech is the physical production of certain sounds and combinations of sounds which when uttered together make a word that communicates meaning. It combines our understanding of language (receptive language) with our ability to produce sound (expressive language) in order to communicate intentions, questions, and information. Speech is only a tiny part of how people communicate. Has anyone ever said to you, "It isn't what you said that upset me but the WAY that you said it?" We communicate as much with our body language, our smiles or frowns, and the tone of our voices as we do by speech.

Our goal is to enrich our children's language experiences as much as possible so that they can more fully communicate with their world. Chapter 2 will explain the process of developing language in young children.

Two

Language Development In Children

As children grow, their physical and mental abilities develop to handle more complex skills. You can see this in an infant absorbed with a rattle, a two-year-old playing with sandbox toys, or a five-year-old building an intricate structure with blocks. Each is playing

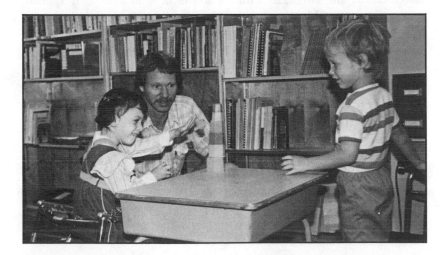

Language Development In Normally Hearing Children

Vocal Play ◄─►	Babbling ◄─►	Jargon ◄─►	Imitation ◄─►
0 months	6 mos.	12 mos	18mos.
	1 word	3 words	22 words

Phrases ◄─►	Sentences/ ◄─► Questions	Paragraphs ◄─►	Nearly Correct ◄─► Grammar
24 mos.	3 years	4 years	5 years
272 words	896 words	1870 words	2289 words

Full Command of English
6 years
2568 words

Vocabulary numbers taken from Diagnostic Methods in Speech Pathology, p. 192.
Samples taken from children of average IQ.

within a different range of abilities that is appropriate for his growth at that age.

Language ability also develops over time. From a child's first "mama" or "dada" through complete phrases and sentences made up of several words, an amazing amount of language development occurs. Like other areas, language development varies tremendously between children.

When you are playing with your child, you are striving to help him increase his language skills. Parents of children with special needs often ask, "What is considered 'normal' language development so I can gauge my child's progress?" Figure 1 shows stages of language development in children. Remember, there is a very wide range of what is considered "normal" development and there could be a wide variation in your child's language skills.

Parents, teachers, therapists, and other specialists want to be able to determine the level where your child is functioning. His development in areas such as fine motor, gross motor, thinking, receptive language, expressive language, and speech are tested to determine his strengths and weaknesses. Extensive studies by experts have established ages where most of the children tested acquired each skill. By comparing your child with these norms, the approximate age at which your child is functioning can be found.

This is called a *developmental age*. Since there is great variation among children, most tests will give a range from the lowest age where this skill is acquired to the highest age where almost every child tested had the skill. This developmental range is the most accurate way to find where your child is functioning at this time.

For parents of children with special needs, development can be complicated. Often these children are a mosaic of different developmental levels. A child may have six-year-old gross motor skills, two-year-old fine motor skills, and another level in language development. Deciding where your child currently is *developmentally* in his language skills can be a little tricky.

We have prepared summaries of different developmental ages that emphasize language development. Their ranges will enable you to determine your child's current level of language development. We have also included physical development so that you can have a clear picture of your child's development overall. Remember, these developmental ages are general outlines only. No two children are alike. Far more important than comparing your child's behavior to other children within the same range is to compare your child's behavior, accomplishments, and progress with himself. It is not critical that your child reach any given stage by a certain age. Quality of development – not just quantity – should be your goal.

In working with your child with developmental delays in language, use his developmental age and not his actual age. For instance, he may be chronologically twenty-four months old, but his language may have developed to a twelve-month-old level. In your work with him, use the language developmental age of twelve months. He will function best at his developmental age and you do not want to frustrate him by working beyond his capabilities.

Developmental Ages

This section summarizes developmental ages of children during the first five years of life. This information will help you decide what language developmental age best fits your child now so you can choose appropriate language activities.

One way for you to decide which toys your child will enjoy is to see which category lists the largest number of skills your child has acquired. This level should be close to his developmental age. Using toys from this category should insure that you and your child will benefit from the activities presented. Our selections should not limit you but should be used as a guide. Choose any toy that you think he will enjoy playing with and learn from.

Birth To Three Months

A newborn is primarily interested in his most basic needs for food, comfort, and love. He spends most of his day being nourished, being kept clean, and being loved. During this time he is developing an understanding of trust and warmth from those who care for him.

Language Development

During his first few weeks of life, your baby is most likely to communicate only through crying. The people taking care of him will soon be able to tell what his different cries mean. Is he hungry? Is he wet? Is he tired? Does he want company? Each of these cries has a different tone to it which can be understood easily in a short time. In a few weeks your baby adds cooing, squealing, and gurgling to his repertoire. You can see that he enjoys making all these different sounds as you talk to him, play with him, tickle him, and make those favorite silly faces that we enjoy making with little babies.

The little noises that infants make in these first months are called *vocal play*. Most infants will engage in vocal play. The sounds are vowel-like and can vary in loudness as well as in the pitch of high and low sounds. In these first few months babies often make sounds that are heard in languages other than their own. An American baby might produce an inflectional tone of an Asian language, a guttural sound from a Germanic language, or a tongue click from an African dialect. Because these sounds are not reinforced by the sounds he hears around him, he quickly stops playing with them and focuses more on the sounds that are reinforced in his own language. It is in this way that babies begin to learn to speak their native language.

Physical Development

During the first three months of life, you may see that your infant is developing an awareness of his sense of touch. You can get a response from him by rubbing his hands, arms, legs, and feet with smooth, scratchy, fuzzy, and soft materials. By the third month, he will be able to hold onto objects and will enjoy rattles and stuffed animals.

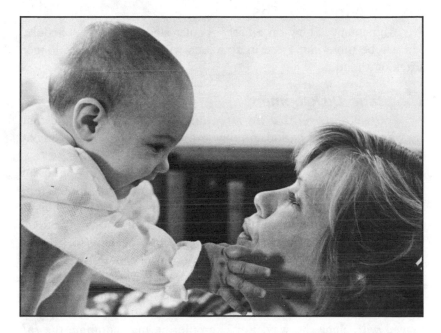

Three To Six Months

Your baby is now becoming more active and is awake for longer periods of time. He's ready for more play time with you. Instead of spending most of your time just caring for your newborn, now you can increase both the amount of time you spend playing with him and can focus this play more on his language development.

Language Development

Around the fourth month, we begin to hear more of the consonant sounds emerging in his vocal play. He will practice with sounds that use only his lips such as /m/b/p/ as well as sounds using other parts of his mouth, such as his tongue, which produce /t/g/l/.

Physical Development

Your baby is able now to grasp and hold onto things and will enjoy rattles, stuffed animals, and objects that he can explore with his hands like those textured rattles and animals you bought when he was a newborn. He is able to reach out for things and bring them to his mouth to explore them.

Six To Nine Months

Your infant is now on a fairly regular sleep and play schedule. He will be more interested in activities with you and awake longer to enjoy them.

Language Development

You will discover that his attention span is increasing and that he will enjoy longer periods of play and longer periods of looking at books and pictures with you.

Beginning at about six months, your baby's random sounds of vocal play will begin to become repetitive. You'll hear more combinations of sounds that he will repeat over and over again. This is called *babbling*. You may even hear some combinations of sounds that resemble actual words. They rarely hold meaning for him at this point. Gradually, at around eight months of age, these babbling sounds get more refined and begin to represent words to your baby. Around this time, you will hear his first true word, which will usually be a combination of consonant and vowel sounds that he has played with along the way. For example, he may combine the /a/ and /m/ sounds to produce "mama," or may combine /a/ with /b/ to produce "baba."

Physical Development

He is becoming more physically active and may be ready to crawl very soon. By the end of this time range, he may well be crawling along. He can sit up by himself, which makes him more available for different games that you can play. His fine motor skills are becoming more refined and he is able to pick up things using his thumb to help him. He'll be able to pick up blocks and help you in stacking them and in knocking them down! He'll enjoy stacking rings, but at first he will be more interested in taking them off than he will be in putting them back on.

By the end of this time period, he will be pulling himself up to a standing position, so be sure to raise the sides of the crib and put away that crystal vase!

Nine To Twelve Months

Language Development

As he moves along toward his first birthday, you will see a dramatic rise in your baby's comprehension (receptive language). He will enjoy playing games of "Show me." "Show me your eyes." "Where's the kitty?" "Can you find your ball?" He will enjoy showing off how much he understands and may even try to imitate some of the key words he hears you say.

His attention span is still increasing and he will enjoy listening to books, records, and tapes. He may even be able to point to some known objects in the books as you tell him the names.

Physical Development

By now you've noticed how very physically active your baby is. He will be holding on and walking around furniture. He may even strike out on his own and walk by himself. He will enjoy active outdoor play. Make sure that his play area is fenced in or that you are with him all the time. He may be scooting around but he has no idea of danger at this time. He is able to roll a ball with two hands and if he is standing alone by this age, he may even be able to kick it as well. Balls are fun and a great way to encourage physical agility.

His fine motor skills are developing and he is able to pick things up, put them into containers, and gleefully dump them out again. We have seen babies do this over and over for incredibly long periods of time. He is able to manipulate small switches, dials, and slides. He is able to clap his hands together and will enjoy imitating you in pat-a-cake type games.

Twelve To Fifteen Months

Language Development

By now there is much more babbling going on with many sounds strung together into phraselike and sentencelike series. This babbling will have tone and inflection and many people say "If I just knew what language he was speaking...." This phase is called *jargoning*. You will occasionally hear a word tossed in among all of his singsong jargoning.

Physical Development

One of the play skills your toddler will find most interesting is turning "dumping" into "pouring." If he has been walking and is steady, he will now be able to walk sideways and backward and will enjoy walking with pull toys as well as push toys.

Up until now you have been rolling a ball to him. Since he is now steadily standing, he will be able to throw the ball to you. He probably will not be able to catch it yet but he will enjoy kicking and chasing it.

His fine motor skills are well developed enough now that he can turn the pages of a book and do other fine motor activities.

Fifteen To Eighteen Months

Your baby's imagination is developing and he will like playing with toys that are representational of his world. He will enjoy acting out many scenes that he sees in his own life.

Language Development

Jargoning continues while words develop. By eighteen months, you'll be able to distinguish more and more recognizable words mixed in the jargon. If you are keeping a list of words for which he has true meanings, you'll probably find that he says somewhere around 22-25 words. These are certainly not absolute numbers —some children may say more and some fewer—but this number is an average for an eighteen-month-old baby.

Physical Development

During this stage, your child is able to climb stairs and expand his world on his own. He now has the physical abilities he needs to indulge his curiosity. He will explore your home inside and out. Be sure to provide a safe environment for him.

Eighteen To Twenty-Four Months

At this age your child's interest in books continues and now he is able to "read" the pictures himself. He will enjoy "reading" to you out of homemade books that you may have made for him earlier. He can even help select pictures for new books.

Language Development

At this age, your toddler enjoys imitating your words, tones, and actions. Now is a great time for finger plays and games like peek-a-boo and pat-a-cake. If you check the language development chart, you will see a dramatic rise in the number of words your little one is now able to use. An average number of words that he might be using is about 272 by twenty-four months of age. We share this number with you so you are aware of the vast number of things he can identify by name. He also will be combining these words into short phrases. You'll hear him say–"Bye bye car"–"Daddy go work". You'll also hear many incorrect grammatical combinations such as "Tommy falled down" or "car go me." You'll begin to hear pronouns being used although he will still refer to himself by name most of the time. His pronunciation of words and phrases can often be very hard to understand.

Physical Development

Your young child is probably very active at this stage. He is walking steadily, running constantly, climbing, and now adds jumping to his repertoire.

His fine motor skills are developed to the point where he can open and close containers. He will be able to place puzzle pieces if there is one piece for each space.

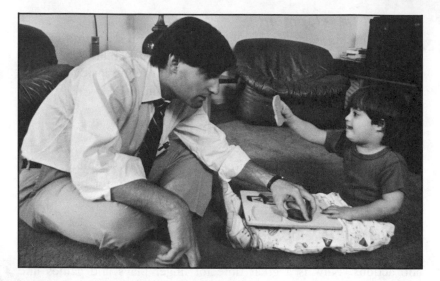

Twenty-Four To Thirty-Six Months

Language Development

This is a fascinating time for you and your child in many ways. Language development is certainly one of the most exciting things happening during this year. This is the year where the phrases of 2-3 words turn into sentences of 4-5 words. The sentences then turn into questions. This is the year of "why," "what," and "where." Sometimes these questions are really for the purpose of gaining information and sometimes your child just enjoys hearing himself talk.

You can expect your child to make many errors in the use of words and how they fit into sentences. He really does not understand the rules of grammar yet. He will also mispronounce many sounds at this age, and for the next few years. Figure 2 shows you when each of the speech sounds usually develops.

Physical Development

By this age he has many of his large motor skills under control. He may be able to pedal a trike but more likely he will push with his feet on the ground. He will probably discover the low-seated plastic Big Wheels that children enjoy at this age.

His fine motor skills continue to develop and he will be able to play with interlocking block systems to create endless imaginative

FIGURE 2

Earliest Ages At Which Sounds Were Correctly Produced, In the Word Positions Indicated, by 75% of 208 Children

Consonants	Beginning Position	Middle Position	End Position
m	2	2	3
n	2	2	3
ng	6	3	*
p	2	2	4
b	2	2	3
t	2	5	3
d	2	3	4
k	3	3	4
g	3	3	4
r	5	4	4
l	4	4	4
f	3	3	3
v	5	5	5
th (vl)	5	*	*
th (v)	5	5	*
s	5	5	5
z	5	3	3
sh	5	5	5
h	2	*	*
wh	5	*	*
w	2	2	*
y	4	4	*
ch	5	5	4
j	4	4	6

Vowels and Dipthongs	Age
ee (beet)	2
i (bit)	4
e (bed)	3
a (cat)	4
u (cup)	2
ah (father)	2
aw (ball)	3
oo (foot)	4
oo (boot)	2
u-e (mule)	3
o-e (coke)	2
a-e (cake)	4
i-e (kite)	3
oy (boy)	3

* not tested

Figure 2 (continued)

Consonant Blends	Age	Consonant Blends	Age
pr	5	-ks	5
br	5	sl	6
tr	5	sw	5
dr	5	tw	5
kr	5	kw	5
gr	5	ngk	4
fr	5	ngk	5
thr	6	-mp	3
pl	5	-nt	4
bl	5	-nd	6
kl	5	spr-	5
gl	5	spl-	5
fl	5	str-	5
-ld	6	skr-	5
-lk	5	skw-	5
-lf	5	-ns	5
-lv	5	-ps	5
-lz	5	-ts	5
sm-	5	-mz	5
sn-	5	-nz	5
sp-	5	-ngz	5
st-	5	-dz	5
-st	6	-gz	5
sk-	5		

* Powers, Margaret Hall, "Functional Disorders of Articulation/Symptomotology and Etiology." In *Handbook of Speech Pathology and Andiology,* edited by Lee Edward Travis, p. 842.

designs. He is comfortable handling puzzle pieces and enjoys showing off his skills.

Thirty-Six To Forty-Eight Months

During this year, most young children are involved with other children on a regular basis. Your child will continue to be very active both in and out of doors with playmates and alone.

Language Development

As your child's world begins to expand beyond your doors, new people will be adding to his receptive language. He will begin to have new playmates in the neighborhood and at his preschool or daycare center. He will pick up new and different words and phrases from them.

You will notice that he is able to tell you more complicated stories about things that happen to him when you aren't around. He can tell you about his activities at school and about his play with friends outside.

One disturbing development in his expressive language that may happen during this year may be the occurrence of *nonfluency*. Nonfluency usually happens like this: Your child has many things he wants to tell you. They are all very important to him and often he is overwhelmed with excitement at telling you about them. His thoughts may come so quickly that his oral muscles may not be able to keep up with the speed of his thinking.

Give your child time and attention during these moments. Do *not* comment about his nonfluency. Do *not* suggest that he calm down and slow down. Do *not* give him the words he is stumbling over. The problem will usually evaporate in time if you do not focus on it. There are differing opinions about the subject of nonfluency in young children but it is our opinion that the less you make of it the better. A note of caution: If the nonfluency continues past age five or if your child develops some other behaviors to go along with it such as a nervous twitch, or stamping his foot as he is talking, or any other involvement of other parts of his body, you will want to have an evaluation done by a speech pathologist, a trained professional familiar with the normal patterns of language development in young children.

It is important for you to note that we call this "nonfluency." You may want to call it stuttering or stammering but these are loaded terms and do not accurately represent what is happening at this stage. What you actually hear is a nonfluency and this happens for normal and natural reasons.

Physical Development

His fine motor skills are developed enough that he can hold small markers for games. He will begin pedaling his tricycle, may enjoy pulling and being pulled in a wagon, and will use playground equipment such as swings and slides. An outdoor sandbox is a great toy and can be used with his cars and toy people to act out play scenes.

Forty-Eight To Sixty Months

Language Development

He will be using well over two thousand words by the time he is five. He will be talking in complete paragraphs and you will begin to see that most of his grammatical errors have straightened themselves out. He may still have a few errors in the speech sounds themselves but if he is generally easy to understand by you and others outside your family, you do not need to concern yourself with these few errors. Complete sentences and phrases continue to proliferate.

Physical Development

By the time your child is five, he will be able to walk on a line, hop on one foot for about ten seconds, jump over a rope, and catch a large ball when you bounce it to him.

No time of life is as full of as much development and growth as the period from birth to age five. It is almost magic for parents—including parents of children with developmental delays—to observe as their children grow, change, and learn. But parents of children with a delay in language development need to know what may cause this. The knowledge of language development that you have learned is your foundation for understanding problems that may occur in this area.

Possible Causes Of
Language Delay In Children

We have talked about how receptive language, expressive language, and speech evolve in a child who is moving along the developmental milestones in a normal fashion. How does this differ if there are developmental delays of one kind or another? There have been volumes written on this subject and it is not the intent of this book to focus in detail on various disabilities. We do, however, describe a variety of developmental disabilities that may have an effect on language development.

In reading about each of those disabilities, bear in mind that each child is unique and his abilities are unlike any other child's even if he shares the same generic label of a particular disability. We have seen profoundly retarded children who have not been expected to walk or talk do both under guidance from professionals and parents who believe in their potential. But while we need to keep our expectations high, we should not close our eyes to the obvious. In spite of our greatest efforts, some of our children may never achieve the level that we would like to see for them. Reach for the stars but make them stars you can see, not just hope to see. Rejoice in what your child is able to achieve, in the potential he is able to realize.

Cognitive Ability

The relationship of intelligence to language development is a most complex issue. Once again, it should never be assumed that a "low IQ" is an absolute predictor of language development. Many articles have been written about the accuracy of IQ measurements and there is no clear-cut evidence that an IQ is a very good predictor of anything, especially language development. When we speak of an average IQ, we do not mean that a child with an average IQ should only be expected to acquire average language development. We know that experiences, exposure to interesting and exciting vocabulary, as well as personal motivation, can enhance anyone's language development.

If, however, we are talking about children who have been diagnosed as having specific disorders such as Down syndrome, brain injury, or other conditions that can cause mental retardation, then we know that language development will be slower than for children of the same age without these conditions. This does not mean, however, that we stop speaking to this child or stop giving him enriching language experiences. Just the opposite is true: this child needs more language stimulation than other children. Remember that receptive language must come first, and if he has nothing to talk about, it is certain that he will not have expressive language.

The child with mental retardation will acquire language at a slower rate than a child of average or higher intelligence, but in most cases he will acquire language. It will be necessary for you to work at the developmental level of your child rather than at his chronological age. When you read our chapter on toys, find a toy that fits with your child's developmental age rather than his chronological age. You will both derive more pleasure from the play this way than if you try to interest him in something that is beyond his abilities.

Physical Disabilities

Speech is the goal for every child. However, it is only one form of expressive language. If we give a child a rich background of receptive language, but, because of some physical disability, he does not have the ability to form sounds through speech, it may be possible for him to learn language and to communicate through sign language, communication boards, or other visual systems. Today's technology allows people who are unable to verbalize to communicate. Computers have voice synthesizers as well as the ability to communicate visually with another person. Speech is a small part of communication.

A child who has severe physical disabilities may be delayed in his language development because so much of his time is spent working with his physical limitations that he simply doesn't have the time to spend enriching his language. He may require many hospitalizations which reduce the amount of time that he is in his own home. This can produce stress for him as well as for you. Neither of you may have much energy left for playing with toys or games. Additionally, he may not have the physical ability to manipulate toys in ways that will facilitate playing. If the physical problems that your child has interfere with the small muscles which are necessary for the production of speech, you may find that he has excellent receptive language and yet is physically unable to produce the sounds necessary for speech. It is at this point that you must find alternative ways of communication: sign systems, communication boards, computers and other new technology.

Environment

Many studies have compared how children are raised in families with how they are raised in institutions. Looking first at families, it is often, but not, always found that firstborn children begin to speak sooner than their siblings. This is probably because parents may have the time for more interaction when they only have one child. Subsequent children may be given less parental time. On the other hand, there are equally as many studies that have shown that children in large families talk early as well because they have many more people to interact with and often learn more from their brothers and sisters than they do from their parents. The key, of course, is that someone must be talking to the child so that receptive language can be built.

By contrast, children who are raised in institutions where there are more children than adults are often delayed in language development. These findings have had a profound impact on modern daycare centers. More and more centers are making it a priority to have low adult-child ratios and to encourage language development among the children through stimulating activities. These studies underscore one important point: It is essential to language development to provide children–particularly children with special needs–with a rich receptive language environment.

The language a child hears in the environment should closely resemble the language that will be used in the school he attends. This has raised questions about bilingual families. Current research shows that children can learn both languages–the native family language and the one he hears in the environment. It is true that these children may have more catching up to do when they enter the school environment than those children who speak the same language as the instructional one. In no circumstances should parents who speak a different language speak no language to their child for fear of him having problems in school. If the child has a rich receptive language background, regardless of the language, he will be more successful than if he has no receptive language at all.

Sensory Deficits

Children who have hearing impairments or visual impairments are at a disadvantage in learning language. Visual impairments limit what the child can actually experience for himself but in no way limit the input that an adult can supply to overcome that deficit. Colors, though difficult to describe to someone who has never seen them, can be adequately described in terms of how they relate to objects the child knows or can learn about that remain constant. For example, a lemon is yellow, apples are red, and potatoes are brown. Use consistent color references often with your visually impaired child. Using these other senses for the visually impaired can help them to understand, if not entirely know, the concepts of things they cannot see.

Hearing impairment, on the other hand, almost always produces a deficit in receptive language. Without the ability to hear a spoken language, it is very difficult to build a receptive base of language in the critical early language years. Many volumes have been written on the "best" way to convert spoken language into visual language. There is no clear "best" way. You will have to explore to find the best way for your child.

Whatever your child's special needs may be, it is important that you determine the nature of his language delay as early as possible. The earlier you find out how he is delayed, the earlier you can begin to help him catch up. Use the following checklist to help you determine if your child has a problem in his language development.

Recognizing Speech And Language Problems Early

If your child exhibits any of the following fifteen problems, you should consider consulting a speech pathologist to evaluate your child's language development.

1. Your child is not talking by the age of two years.

2. His speech is largely unintelligible after the age of three.

3. He is leaving off many beginning consonants after the age of three.

4. He is still not using two to three word sentences by the age of three.

5. Sounds are more than a year late in appearing in his speech according to their developmental sequence.

6. He uses mostly vowel sounds in his speech.

7. His word endings are consistently missing after the age of five.

8. His sentence structure is noticeably faulty at the age of five.

9. He is embarrassed and disturbed by his speech.

10. He is noticeably nonfluent after the age of six.

11. He is making speech errors other than /wh/ after the age of seven.

12. His voice is a monotone, too loud, too soft, or of a poor quality that may indicate a hearing loss.

13. His voice quality is too high or too low for his age and sex.

14. He sounds as if he were talking through his nose or as if he has a cold.

15. His speech has abnormal rhythm, rate, and inflection after the age of five.

This was reprinted from: *Teach Your Child To Talk,* by David Pushaw, published by CEBCO Standard Publishing, 104 5th Ave., New York, NY.

Assessment

If you have been concerned that your child has a delay in language development, you will want to have an assessment done by a trained speech pathologist. An assessment is a complete evaluation of the speech and language skills that your child has acquired. His strengths and needs will be determined which will be used in planning how to help him.

You should ask your pediatrician if she can recommend someone to do this assessment. If she doesn't know of a speech pathologist in your area, you can contact the American Speech Language Hearing Association (ASHA) at 10801 Rockville Pike, Rockville, MD 20852. You can call collect to the Helpline at ASHA by calling 1/301/897–8682 (Voice or TTY). This association will be able to give you names of certified speech clinicians in your area. If you are unable to make this contact for any reason, try your local college or university and ask if they have a department which trains future speech pathologists. They will be able to refer you to someone for an evaluation.

Taking A History

When you come for your child's assessment, the speech pathologist will want a complete history of your child's s growth up to now. If you have kept baby records, bring them with you to help you remember important milestone events in your child's life. If you have medical information about his special needs, you will want to bring this along with you as well. The more information you can provide about your child, the more the clinician will be able to help you determine where your child might be in his language development.

Testing

Clinicians use a variety of assessment tools to help determine where your child's language development is. Some tests will ask *you* for information about your child while others directly ask the child to respond to various questions which will indicate his understanding and expression of language.

Testing Receptive Language

Your child's receptive abilities will be tested by asking him to point out objects or pictures when they are named or to choose between sets of pictures in response to a word or group of words that is presented by the therapist. In one test, for instance, your child will be shown a small doll and will be asked to point to various facial and body parts. "Where is the dolly's nose, eyes, ears, etc.?" His responses will be recorded on a testing sheet which will later be used to determine his language development level.

In all of these tests the questions get increasingly more difficult, and your child will begin to be unable to respond. The clinician will keep testing to reach the level where your child is no longer able to respond. This will indicate the upper level of his understanding. It will let the clinician know what level to focus on when working with him later on.

Testing Expressive Language

Almost all of the language tests that are used with young children use objects or pictures to encourage children to respond in certain expected ways. For example, on the Structured Photographic Expressive Language Test (SPELT), your child will be shown pictures of modern everyday situations. He will be asked questions such as "What is the girl wearing?" The expected response is, "A dress" or "A red dress." These items are structured so that all the parts of language are tested. Single nouns, plural nouns, possessive nouns, possessive pronouns, and so on, are all tested. This and other language tests will give the clinician a good idea of areas where your child might need help and where his strengths are.

Oral Mechanism Exam

The speech clinician will want to check inside your child's mouth. She will want to check the roof of your child's mouth (palate) to see that everything is formed correctly. She will check the size and movement of your child's tongue and see the alignment of his teeth, lips, and jaw. All of these parts of the mouth area are involved in the production of speech. Your child's ability to control drooling will also be examined as well as the tone of the muscles in the mouth area.

Speech Sounds

If your child is talking at all, the clinician will want to systematically check to see which sounds he pronounces correctly and which he has difficulty with. Again, pictures will be used for the stimulus. The pictures will be of objects that show the sound wherever they generally occur in words. For example, for the sound "B" the pictures might be:

beginning: bed
middle: baby
end: tub

Your child may have some omissions or substitutions of sounds. Their significance will depend on your child's age.

To ensure a complete picture of your child's language development, be sure to tell the clinician of your child's language experiences at home. Your input is important for a complete assessment.

Immediately after the evaluation of your child, the speech clinician will be able to tell you a few specific things that she noticed. Usually, however, you will need to wait longer for a final and more complete report. Be ready to return to review the findings and to follow through on the suggestions that the clinician will make.

Conclusion

Children with language development delays are still like other children. They will go through most if not all of the language development stages that all children go through. With your special child, however, more effort may be needed to help him achieve language skills like other children.

Understanding language development in children is essential to understanding where your child might have a problem. Knowing what some causes of language delay are can help you understand your own child's particular problem. Finally, an assessment by a speech and language pathologist can identify the type of language delay your child has and help you get to work to overcome that delay. That *work* is in reality *play* for your child, and understanding how your child will approach that *work/play* is vital to teaching your child language skills. The next chapter explains this fascinating world of child play.

Three

Playing And Learning

Why Play Is Important

In our technological society where we are busy trying to cure cancer, solve our nation's problems about nuclear energy, and live in harmony with countries of clashing political viewpoints, can we allow our children to relax, have fun, and play? Of course we can!

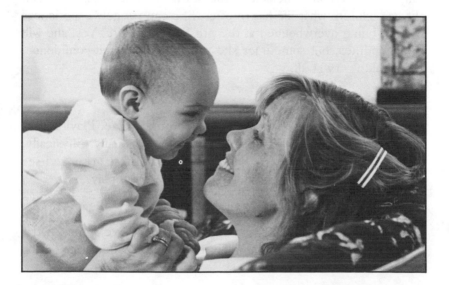

More than that, we should encourage them to play. Why? Because play is important for children; it is a way for them to learn.

It is through play that children learn about the world around them. While playing, children test ideas, ask questions, and come up with answers. For instance, in playing with nesting blocks, your child learns about size relationships—she learns that smaller blocks fit inside larger ones. She learns cause and effect as she builds her blocks higher and higher until they come crashing down. When her blocks come tumbling down, she can link that to the world of experiences and ideas by using the language we are teaching her.

Play begins in infancy. There are simple games you and your baby play as you interact during feeding time. Your baby sucks on the bottle or breast and if you pull the milk source away, the baby will suck harder, wiggle her toes and fingers, and give you the message that she wants her bottle back. Trading smiles and fake coughs is another early game played between infants and parents. Through these basic games, your baby learns that her actions have an effect on the people around her. She learns early basic ways to control those larger people in her life. As she gains more and more control over her environment, her idea of who she is and what she can accomplish develops in a positive way. She learns self-confidence as she sees that what she does influences what happens to her. She can use this vision of herself as the sturdy foundation from which she can explore what life has to offer. She can try new experiences without being overwhelmed at the prospect of failure. Yes, she will fail sometimes, but sometimes she won't. Without self-confidence, she wouldn't try at all.

The Value Of Play

Play time is more than just "fooling around" time. Playing with toys with your child can help her develop emotionally, physically, socially, and cognitively. We'll look at each of these areas and see how you can help her grow in these ways through play.

Emotional Development

If your child has a language delay, she may have some frustrations to work out. It is emotionally difficult for children not to be able to adequately communicate their needs. The inability to communicate is hard on any child, but when you add a handicapping condition with its special needs, the frustration level can be almost intolerable. By carefully watching her play you will be able to see areas of frustration that she may have. She will give you hints by the way she handles her dolls, the actions she has play-people perform, or her reactions to stories you read her.

Through play your child can work out some of her feelings of anxiety or concern. If, for example, she sees a physical therapist twice a week and these visits cause her discomfort, you might want to structure a play situation with her where the toy "therapist" comes to the house to help the little girl feel stronger in her legs, arms, or wherever the difficulties are. Your child can then work out some of her feelings during this play time and you can point out what is positive about what the "therapist" is doing.

In a similar way, if your child had a disagreement with a friend a little while ago, you might want to structure a play situation where you help her work out a solution to the problem. This will keep you from interfering when the friend is there, yet give you a way to show your child what to do the next time she is in a similar situation.

You can encourage positive emotional growth in your child when you interact through play. She will see that you are interested in spending time with her and that you respond to her needs. Children need to feel loved and valued in order to grow. The time you spend with her reinforces her vision of herself as a person who is worthy of your time and love.

As your child gets older, she does not lose her emotional need for some control of her world. By playing with your child, you can allow her to have the control in play that she may not be able to have in real life. If we go back to our example of the physical therapist, you can allow your child to have one of her toy people refuse to see the "therapist," whereas in real life she cannot refuse. She will learn that she can control some areas of her life but not others.

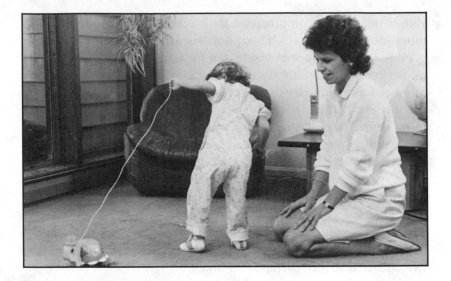

Physical Development

Your child may be language delayed, but it is very possible that her physical skills are right on par. This will be very encouraging to you as well as to her. She can do things with her hands and feet that perhaps she just is not able to do with language. She will feel confident if you pick up on those physical strengths that she does have and encourage language development around them. For example, you can ask her to shake her rattle. As she does this, you can say, "Good! You are doing a great job of shaking the rattle." You can emphasize specific sounds like **sh** and encourage her to imitate you.

You can stress how well she plays with her toys. You can remind her that she is getting so big that now she can hold the block in one hand. Toys can be a way to give her a sense of pride in what she can accomplish physically.

If your child also has physical limitations, you will want to make sure to use toys that she can handle and to encourage her by making adaptations in the toys. For example, if she has small motor difficulties and loves to play board games, you might want to add velcro to the board and the bottoms of the markers so that she can easily move her marker along and play the game.

Social Development

The social play of children passes through three stages. At first the very young child plays alone. She does not like to interact with playmates her own age although she will interact with you. Gradually she will move into parallel play where she will play nicely alongside a friend doing similar kinds of things but not involving each other. The final stage of social play is where the children play together with each contributing something to the play situation. If your child has a language delay, this could be the stage that presents some difficulties for her. By the time children are ready to engage in social play, they need language to communicate ideas. You will then see that you can use your play time to give her the vocabulary that she will need in order to play with her friends.

Your child learns from you that sharing her toys is a fine way for you to play together and that each of you can take a turn. She learns that when her friends come over it is okay to share with them and wait her turn. These are difficult skills for children to learn, but you can practice with her when you are alone. Through imaginative play, you can play out a situation that you had seen that afternoon in the park where another child was not being very nice to your child. You can show your child how to be sensitive to another person's feelings through this kind of pretend play.

Many more children today are exposed to men and women in nontraditional career roles. They will see more women doctors than you did when you were growing up. They will see more men in jobs that previously only women seemed to perform. Your daughter can use her toy cars and trucks to play mechanic while your son is using the play kitchen to fix lunch. Playing with these toys in nontraditional ways encourages your child to accept society's move away from stereotyping. This is another example of the way that toys can represent our world to our children.

Cognitive Development

There are four stages of cognitive development in children. How does knowing them help you interact with your child and her toys? Your child's ability to think, understand, and eventually reason things out is a dynamic process. With each new toy, game, or experience that you introduce, your child is taking in all the information and knowledge her brain is capable of assimilating depending on her level of development. Although each stage is separate, they are all dependent on each other for success. With the exact same toy, game, or sample dialogue provided in this book, your child can extract from it what she is capable of understanding' at any given developmental point in time. Later on she will derive something different from the same toy. As a parent you can help challenge your child's ability to her potential within each stage as well as looking ahead to what comes next.

The first stage, which is the *sensorimotor stage*, is roughly from birth to two years of age. Your child will be learning about her environment through her muscles and her senses. By watching, hearing, touching, and feeling she will learn about things around her. You will be giving her language for things that she sees in her daily life such as water, spoon, and ball. She will experience them by touching, seeing, and physically interacting with them.

The second stage, which is the *representational stage*, occurs from two to seven years of age. Your child will begin to be able to represent things by using symbols instead of the real thing. It is during this stage that her language will develop the most.

The third stage, which is the *concrete operations stage* and occurs from age seven to eleven, is when your child is able to think through a situation without having to actually act it out. She is able to see the consequences of her actions and think about what may happen before it actually happens.

The fourth stage, which is the *formal operations stage* and begins around age eleven, is where you will find that your child is really able to do serious problem solving. She is able to reason with abstract thoughts and does not need to have the concrete observation to depend on.

As a child progresses through these stages of cognitive development her ability to play will become increasingly sophisticated to the point that it ceases to be merely "play" and begins to resemble concerted problem solving, exploration, and analysis. Let's look at how play with a ball might change through each of these stages.

In the earliest sensorimotor stage, a parent would want to expose his child to the idea that the toy they are playing with is called a ball. "Look Tyrone, this is a ball. It is round. It is hard. Can you hold it? Can you roll it to Mommy? Look. Mommy can catch the ball. Now Daddy will help you catch it. Let's see if we can throw it way up in the sky."

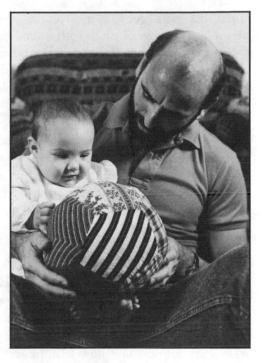

At such an early stage in infancy, a child might not understand any of the words Mother is saying. However, the child is receiving an invaluable language learning experience. Through Mother's words, Tyrone can begin to understand what the word ball really means—what it feels like, how it can be thrown and caught, that it is round and smooth, and that it moves apart from his hand when he lets go of it, and that it can land in his lap when someone throws it to him.

In the early preoperational stage, the child would understand the game even better based on his earlier, sensorimotor experiences. Tyrone would now begin to understand that when Mom asks, "Do you want to play ball?" it is a give and take, back and forth arrangement that involves the two of them playing together. When Mom asks, "Can you roll it?" or "Can you throw it?" or even, "Can you bounce it?" each word means something different and has a different action associated with it.

Finally, an older preoperational child has often developed enough logic to know that after Mom throws the ball into the air and yells, "Heads UP!" he can go scurrying after it, trying to follow its course so that it will fall straight down into his hands. Although Tyrone would understand this once he enters the preoperational stage, at the younger sensorimotor stage he would not have understood that "what goes up must come down." That's why we don't play a hearty game of catch with a nine-month-old still operating at a sensorimotor level. But that doesn't mean we shouldn't play ball with an infant at all. Earlier action experiences and the language a child learns, set the stage for more complex actions and later learning.

It is easy to see that to a child–especially a child with special needs–"play" is very important. It helps her express herself, develop a positive image of herself, and learn how to interact with the rest of the world. But how can you as her parent involve yourself in her play effectively? The next section discusses using toys to help with language development.

Playing With Toys To Help Develop Language

Toys are how we teach our children about our world and how to live in it. With toys we can teach them how to interact with other people and their environment. And toys can substitute for the world while they are learning how to interact. Playing with toys is particularly important for children who have problems in adjusting to their world.

Since one of the primary goals of play is to teach your child about her world, you need to understand how toys can help her with this goal. When she is young, you represent the world for her. If she can learn to interact with you, she can take those learning experiences with her when she begins interacting with the rest of the world.

Toys Are Interactive

You are your child's first plaything. She reaches out and touches your body as she nurses. She grabs at your nose or Uncle Sonny's glasses. These could be called her first toys. When she grabs you and you respond with a kiss as you remove her hand, the two of you are interacting. She is learning that what she does can have an effect on you. You begin giving her language for her use of these *toys*.

...Be careful, those are Uncle Sonny's glasses. Let's give them back. You touched Mommy's nose– where is your nose? Ouch, it hurts when you pull Mommy's hair. See how gently I stroke your hair...

Because you want to encourage interaction but not at the expense of your nose or glasses, you can substitute toys. You can play with stuffed animals and talk about noses and other facial features. You can hang toys in your child's crib and when she is ready, she can reach out and touch and play with them. The toy will "respond" back as it swings or a small bell rings.

Toys Are Representational

The most significant value of toys may be the way they represent a wider world for your child. Although we encourage you to go on many outings with her to see and experience real life situations, toys can bring these things into your home. You can use toys to prepare children for experiences that are about to happen and then use the toy again after the experience to reinforce what she saw. Let's use the Fisher-Price farm as an example. You have decided that tomorrow 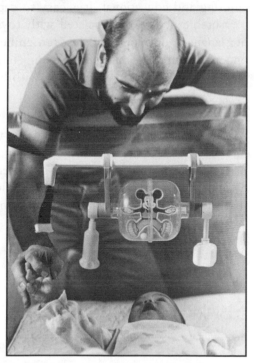 you and your family are going for a ride out to a farm. You can use the Fisher-Price farm to talk about all of the animals that you *will* see on the farm, the buildings that you *will* see on the farm, and the people that you *will* see on the farm. At the farm, you can remind her that the cow is the same color as the toy cow at home or that a real horse is certainly much bigger than the toy horse at home. Later when you have come home from your outing you can go back to the toy farm and talk about what you *saw*. Did you know that you are also teaching verb tenses?

Children with special needs usually spend a lot of time seeing doctors, therapists, and specialists of one kind or another. They are *very* busy children. We don't want you to become one of those parents who is always pushing his child to do one more task, yet you need to spend time to help her develop her language. You can do this through play. You can pick toys that are both fun and can be used to develop her language. The toys in this book are both amusing and educational. It is easy to capitalize on the natural and pleasurable activities associated with toys to help your child with her language development. Just remember that no child learns well under pressure. If you feel that your child has had enough for one session, quit! You can always play with her another time.

Conclusion

In the next section of the book, you will be taking all the information you have just read and putting it to use as you try the dialogues we have written for you. Remember to pick the developmental age that best describes your child, then gather some toys that will work with the dialogues you want to use, and start talking!

Toy Dialogues

Maintaining our children's interest in learning is one of our primary jobs in teaching language. The dialogues have been designed to teach basic language in a variety of ways. We want to send our children off to school as well prepared as possible *and* as excited about learning as they were as infants when they loved our first imitation games. Many an educator has said that if we could maintain the enthusiasm that young children have for learning before they come to school, many of our educational problems would be solved.

How to "Teach" With the Dialogues

As you read the dialogues, you may wonder why there are so many repetitions of key words and concepts. Did you know that a

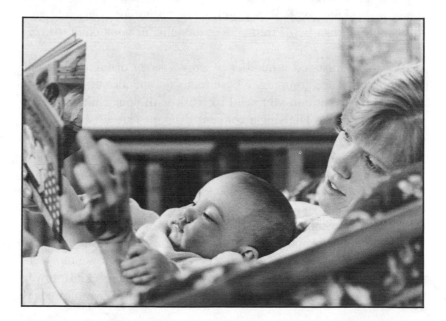

baby must hear thousands of repetitions of a word before he can produce it? As you play with your baby, most of this talking will come naturally.

We have noticed that some people don't talk enough to little children and other people talk on and on never really giving the child a chance to absorb what is being said. As you speak with your child in the short little sentences of the dialogues, you will want to pause ever so slightly between sentences so that he will have the chance to take in what you are saying. If you keep talking on and on, he will only be processing a jumble of meaningless words. As your child gets older, you can increase the length and complexity of your sentences, but still make sure you give him enough time to understand what you are saying. It just takes a little extra time and patience.

Young children have a tremendous need for instant gratification. "I need my bottle NOW!" "No, I want the toy first!" In most situations, including toy play, parents need to remind themselves of the old adage, "A little patience goes a long way."

Children, particularly children with language delays, will benefit more from toy play carried out in a *repetitive* fashion. It may take days, or even weeks, for a child to grasp the concepts of *up* and *down*, or *back* and *forth*. Repetition is not boring for your child and this repetition can be of tremendous benefit for your child's learning.

We have included a number of *single concept* dialogues in each developmental age grouping. These focus on one idea at a time and give you the repetition you need to work with your child stressing just that one idea. The single concept dialogues are of special help to children who may need intensive emphasis in one area.

There are ways to vary the repetition necessary to teach your child. When you are working on the concepts of *back* and *forth*, vary the type and size of the ball. Change the location. With this type of *varied repetition* you and your child will have the advantage of new play activities within the structure he needs in order to learn.

If you want to make play time something your child will look forward to, then you need to be very careful about how you interact with him when the two of you are playing. If your child's tower falls because he has put too many blocks on it, don't give him negative criticism. Toy play should have the same goals as the rest of your interaction with your child—the goal of helping your child develop a good self-image. "Josh, this time you built the tower higher. Isn't it fun to watch all the blocks tumble down when it gets too high?"

Another way to make sure that your child looks forward to his play time with you is to instill in him the joy of learning. This really isn't very hard to do because children are born curious and eager to learn—if the learning is fun. It's up to us to make sure it is. If you sit down with your child and say, "O.K., Josh, today we are going to talk about colors. There are three primary colors. Now repeat after me...." Josh will probably be halfway out of the room before you finish the sentence. Our dialogues are specifically designed to avoid that regimented teaching style. When you use the dialogues, put some enthusiasm into your voice; move around and use gestures. If your child sees that you are having a good time, he will enjoy himself more and find learning fun.

Focus on one toy at a time. Imagine doing a special type of crossword puzzle designed so that all the clues must be examined simultaneously. It would be impossible. This is how your child would feel if you overwhelmed him with a variety of toys and activities all at the same time.

When your child is very young—under two—we suggest that you have as much of your language playtime as you can with him in a high chair. We like to use a high chair because there is a tray to put toys on and the children are at eye level with us. If you can, you might want to have two high chairs in different rooms so that one is associated with eating and the other with playing. If you have only one, that certainly is fine too. Some people also like to use the Sassy Seats that attach to the table. These are fine. The important thing is to be at your child's eye level. That way he is getting additional cues about language from your face. This is particularly important for a hearing impaired child.

Remember to use the actual names of things as much as possible rather than generic terms such as "cars." Talk about station wagons, convertibles, vans, or campers. The richer the language that you put in, the richer the language he will use later on. It is not necessary that he have perfect or even intelligible speech to use rich and powerful language. With the availability of computers today, even the most severely handicapped child can communicate his thoughts.

Try to plan on a few short periods of time each day to use the dialogues. A good time is right after a nap or after snack time. Begin with five or ten minute intervals and gradually increase the amount of time as your child is able to handle it.

You know your child and you will know when he has had enough. Even though we are talking about play time as "teaching" time, it still must be fun and your child must think of it as *play* or he will not stay interested for very long.

Special Considerations

There are a few things to keep in mind for different special needs. If your child is hearing impaired, keep the toy near your mouth so that he can see your lips as you speak to him about the toy. If he is visually impaired, have him hold the toy with you while you describe it. If your child is physically not capable of holding a toy on his own, hold it with him as you describe it to him.

While playing with your language delayed child, there will be many times when you will want to "test" his comprehension by asking him to hand you various objects. This is the earliest way we have of testing whether he understands the meaning of certain words. It is never too early for you to start working on these comprehension skills with your child.

If his speech muscles are impaired due to a physical disability, you may want to teach him sign language so that he can have a way of expressing his needs and wants to you. You may also want to begin teaching him to point to items on a communication board. Even though these are nonverbal methods of communication, they will help him build language skills.

Behavior Management

Behavior management is a major issue if you have a child who is developmentally delayed in any way. You may feel that your child has enough to handle anyway without making his life any more difficult with a lot of rules. If you can look further down the road toward raising a responsible and independent young adult, however, you will realize that catering to his every whim will not help him in the long run. We encourage you to establish consistent guidelines for his behavior and to expect him to abide by them.

During this time, one of your most important roles as a parent will be to teach your child how to behave properly. We've heard parents say how much easier it is just to let their three-year-old walk out of the grocery store with the small package of Lifesavers he's picked up off the shelf than to have a big discipline scene in public. Similarly, it is easier to buy two of every toy for your two children to prevent fighting than it is to teach them to share. We agree wholeheartedly that it is not pleasant or fun to teach discipline to young children. In many instances, it would almost be easier to become invisible and let your child carry on with his antics until he finds a way to resolve things himself.

The fact of the matter is, children do not like it either when they misbehave. It's a frightening feeling for them to be out of control and they need you to set limits for them when they are upset. Believe it or not, deep down inside, your child wants to be a sweet little angel, particularly if his parents value good behavior. If you praise your child as many times for good behavior as you scold him for bad behavior, he will try his hardest to be good. Everyone likes praise.

When he does misbehave, there are many disciplinary methods which work. If you have found one or two which work for you, then simply stick with them. Many parents of three-year-olds are still groping for suitable ways to manage misbehavior. We offer a couple of specific techniques for you here.

One key to good discipline is consistency. This is true for all children, but especially true for your child if he has special needs. If he has a delaying condition which hampers his understanding, you may have to go over concepts many times before your child has a clear understanding of what you mean.

Be firm and clear about which behavior you expect and be as gentle as you can. "Karen, do not grab that toy from Sarah. If you do this again, you may not play together."

If she does grab the toy again, you must stick with what you said and remove her from the play area. She can sit in your designated *time out* area until you feel she is ready to rejoin the other children. Repeat this technique again and again until you feel that she understands the situation.

Another technique that we like is called the *wait technique*. Here's how it works: Let's say that Karen is playing with her friend Rachel. Karen looks over and sees Rachel playing with a Barbie Doll. Of course this looks like more fun than the book that she has been reading. She grabs the Barbie Doll and as they fight over the doll, she hits Rachel. It's time for you to step in. Karen needs to hear the cardinal rule: "There will be no hitting." Under no circumstances should you, the parent, come in and hit your child for hitting the other child! Firmly and gently state the rule, "no hitting," and insist that your child not play until she returns the doll. You can say, "Karen, I'll wait until you're ready." Once she returns the doll, you can then help the two youngsters with the notion of taking turns or trading toys so that each gets a chance to play with the doll.

Social Skills

Many parents of children with special needs feel that neighborhood kids don't want to include their child. One way that you can help bridge that gap is to invite the children to your house and for you to involve yourself some of the time in the play. In this way you can help smooth the road if language gaps get in the way. In these situations, a good rule of thumb is that the maximum number of children who can comfortably play together should equal your child's age in years. Three-year-olds—two playmates, which would be three in total.

We encourage you to start your child in some kind of organized play group or nursery school. This is not to promote the concept of what David Elkind calls the overly educated "hurried child" but rather to expose your child to larger social situations than he would normally receive at home. For the language delayed child, play groups and nursery schools are excellent learning situations, because the children they come in contact with there can provide good speech and language models. Physically delayed children will be exposed to many new opportunities to strengthen their skills under a teacher's careful watch. Overall, a child's impairment is often minimized when he can be a functioning member of the mainstream.

Toy Selection

Just about anything can be a toy! Cardboard boxes, leftover ribbon, spoons—almost anything you can think of. In putting together our list, we had to consider what items would be most easily available for readers in many different areas. Use the toys you want, from wherever you want to get them.

The first consideration for us in selecting toys was safety. Each of the toys that we suggest for a particular developmental age is safe and has been approved by the United States Consumer Product Safety Commission. A list of their criteria is found in Chapter 5 of this book. Then we looked for their suitability for our dialogues, and finally we considered how easily available they would be to consumers around the country. The toys we will use are divided into age categories. Once again, these categories are not absolutes. Many of these toys fit into several age groupings and can be enjoyed by children beyond the ages mentioned here. Children will often use an "old" toy in new and creative ways as their world enlarges and their imaginations develop. In general, the lower age limit is the limit where your child can physically and mentally handle the toy, but the upper limits have no bounds.

Each toy has been selected so that you can interact with your child for the purpose of encouraging and developing expansive and exciting language. This does not mean that your child should not play with the toy alone. He will need time to practice the language skills you have taught him. He may also find new ways to play with the toys that he can show you the next time you play together.

When you first use a toy to "teach" language, it's a good idea not to leave it around to be routinely played with. If you do this, your child may lose interest in your "teaching" activities sooner. Put the toy away safely in a toy chest or on a shelf.

A word here about toy shelves and toy boxes. We recommend shelves for two reasons. One is a safety reason. Often toy boxes have hinged tops, which can close on a child who has crawled inside. Or the lid can slam shut accidentally and perhaps injure your child's head or fingers. The second reason is that toys become lost in a toy box. The ones on the bottom are never seen again as they become buried under layers of other toys. Additionally, they do not have an orderly appearance when they are thrown into a box. We encourage you to use a toy shelf that is sturdy and not very tall. We want your child to be able to reach the shelves himself and not have it topple over on him. The toys should fit easily on the shelves and there should not be room for too many. This way you can have a few toys accessible and keep the others packed away. If you rotate the toys that are on the shelf, your child will maintain his interest in them for a longer period of time.

When working with your language delayed child, you will want to choose a toy that he is physically capable of handling or that you will be able to help him in handling. If he is mentally retarded, then you will want to choose a toy that is appropriate for his developmental age and not necessarily his actual age.

Homemade Toys

We have included at least two homemade toys in each developmental age group. These tested, easy-to-make toys will provide your child with great language learning opportunities. In many cases they are more fun and interesting to play with than many store-bought toys. They can also be less expensive!

Homemade toys give you the opportunity to create and adapt toys to meet your child's own personal needs and preferences. For instance, your child may have a visual impairment in addition to a language delay. You can meet his special needs by printing letters and pictures in extra large, extra bold type.

Conclusion

We hope that you will enjoy using the toy dialogues we have designed and that you will try out the language experiences we suggest. Remember, the toys, dialogues, and techniques you will be using are like the ones professional teachers and therapists use. You will find that as you use the dialogues you will come up with some new ideas of your own that you can expand on from here. Enjoy your play with your child. This is a precious time of sharing experiences and of helping your child grow.

Birth To Three Months Of Age

During your baby's first three months, many new things will be happening. Your whole lifestyle will undergo a change. Your sleeping patterns will change and you may find that you are exhausted. We would like to suggest that you sleep when your baby sleeps and play when he is awake. Save the housecleaning and other chores for another time. Believe it or not, the dirt will still be there waiting for you! Try to avoid getting overtired. You need rest so that you can be available to your baby when he needs you. If you have learned that there is some delaying condition in your newborn, you will especially need this time for your own rest and care. The emotions associated with this discovery can be very exhausting. You may need to add visits to the doctor or special therapists to your daily routine. Try to add in time for yourself too.

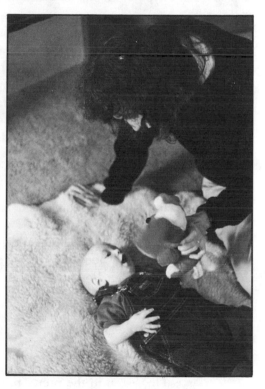

Researchers have spent a lot of time with young babies, looking at what the newborn is most interested in focusing on. Some of these studies have found that the newborn is most interested in bright, primary colors such as red, blue, and yellow. You will see as we describe some of the toys that they are made in these colors. Other researchers have found that newborns really focus best on black and white. We will suggest toys that fit into both categories. Be your own researcher and see what *your* baby likes.

Mobile

A mobile is a colorful and fascinating toy to hang over your baby's changing table, over the crib, or over the kitchen table. We talk about one type of mobile here and then another in the next age category.

Mobiles are available with many different features. Some just swing in the breeze, while others have music boxes attached to them. For our first mobile, we suggest one made by Fisher-Price. This mobile has the animals suspended in such a way that the features of the animal are visible to the infant who is looking *up* at them. Many mobiles have beautiful attachments but the only thing that is visible to the infant is a flat underside! The Fisher-Price mobile has soft attachments shaped like a sheep, a horse, a dog, and a rabbit. Animals are always fascinating to young children because of the sounds that we can imitate. These sounds are usually vowel-like — "aah, aah, ooh, ooh" — and are similar to the earliest sounds that babies make.

A mobile over the changing table gives the newborn something to focus on at a time when he may be feeling uncomfortable and acting fussy. The Fisher-Price mobile has a music box which plays for ten minutes. We suggest that you turn this mobile on before you pick up the infant so that your hands do not have to leave the infant while he is on the changing table. Your conversation, which is, of course, a one-way conversation, will go something like this:

...Oh, listen to the pretty music. Are you wet?
We need to get you into some nice dry pants....

If you know the words to the melody that the mobile is playing, you might want to gently sing the words to it. As the newborn listens to you and the music, he may settle down and stop fussing. Once you have him changed and into fresh clothes, you can spend a few minutes talking about the animals on the mobile.

Point to the animals in turn as you talk about them. You might want to choose a different one each time to talk about.

...Look at the sheep. He has fluffy wool for a
coat. He has four feet, and look at his cute little
tail. Can you see his tail? Let's see. Oh, he also has
two eyes. Look, there are his two eyes. You have
two eyes also just like the sheep. I see his nose. It's
right there. He has a black nose. I see your nose,
too. It's right there. Where is that sheep's mouth?
Oh, I see it. You have a sweet little mouth, too.
What does that sheep say when he talks? He says
'baa-baa.' Let's go now—say 'bye-bye' to the sheep.
Bye sheep. See you later....

The sentences in this conversation are short and you should be
touching the object and relating it to your baby. Gently touching
your baby in the appropriate places reinforces what he is hearing.
We will be talking all through our examples about how to use all
five senses when playing with your baby.

At another time, you will want to talk about the other animals
on the mobile, adding the special characteristics and special sounds
that make a dog different from a horse, sheep, or rabbit. We might
add with the rabbit, that babies will love to watch you wriggle your
nose as bunnies often do. Since newborns love to focus on faces
this will be an added treat.

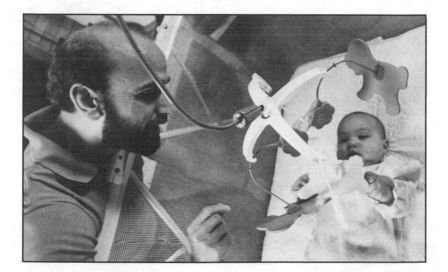

The Fisher-Price mobile is made with bright primary colors which some researchers feel is especially attractive to newborns. As we have said before, you will know which your baby likes. If you are interacting with him and talking about the mobile he will probably like it just fine because what he loves is the interaction.

Stuffed Animal

One of the first toys that newborns usually get as a gift and enjoy interacting with is a stuffed animal. There are so many on the shelves today that any one that is safe and appeals to you will be just fine for the baby to have. We know many children who have so many stuffed animal friends that it is hard to find room in the crib for the baby!

The stuffed animal we recommend is a panda bear because it answers our researchers' finding that newborns focus on objects that are black and white. A stuffed animal offers many new ideas to a newborn. "Stuffed" animals are very soft. They are usually made of a fuzzy kind of material and infants enjoy the stimulation of this texture. Again, research has shown that infants enjoy faces and there are always facial features on stuffed animals. We suggest one that is made in a "face-front" style so that all of the features can be seen at one time. A conversation with your newborn about the Panda Bear may go as follows:

> ...Here's your bear. It's a panda bear. Pandas are black and white. Look, can you see its eyes? It has eyes just like you do. These are your eyes. Can you see the Panda's eyes? Its eyes are black but yours are blue. Jake has blue eyes. Oooh, feel how soft he is....

Stroke your baby's arms, legs, face, and stomach with the bear. Point out all of the features of the bear—his arms, legs, and facial features—and relate them to your infant. Remember from our discussion about language development that he does not understand all of the words that you are using but he will enjoy your voice and, over time, begin to focus on the meaning of what you are saying.

You are the person who "puts in" the language at this time. Without that input, he will not have the vocabulary to use later on.

Rattles

You may receive many rattles as gifts for your newborn. They are generally inexpensive and friends enjoy tying one to the outside of their gifts. It is interesting that this is such a popular toy for a newborn, because babies do not have the coordination to hold a rattle. Nevertheless, *we* can make use of the rattle that you receive as a source of sound and sight stimulation for your infant. Rattles vary in intensity of sound; some are very soft with tiny little beads and others have wooden parts which clap together and are louder and lower in tone. Use them all and see which ones your baby responds to best. During the first month, you may see him respond to the sound of the rattle by blinking his eyes. Later, toward the end of his second month, he will begin to search for the sound if you shake the rattle off to the side of his head. If you do not notice him searching for the rattle, move it slowly around to the front of him until he does focus on it. Then talk to him about the sound and try it again from the side. He may need to play this game a few times before he understands what it is that he is listening for. To stimulate him visually with a rattle, you can hold it in front of his eyes and then very slowly move it off to the side. Talking about the movement of the rattle will help him to focus on it as it moves.

> ...Here's your rattle. Watch, here it goes. Can you follow it? There you go. Here it comes back again....

Your baby should be able to follow a rattle in this way.

As we have said, there are many fine rattles on the market today. One style that we suggest that you look into is a wrist rattle. There are several that are made by Playskool, Fisher-Price, and Chicco. These are soft rattles that go around a baby's wrist. Some attach to themselves with velcro, while others are made of a stretchable terry-type fabric which can go on the baby's wrist. Rattles like these allow your baby to control the production of the sound and to be amused by the sound when it is made involuntarily by his generalized movement. The soft fabric is additional physical stimulation, which is so important to a newborn.

Texture Toys

Toy manufacturers know that infants need stimulation by textured toys. Almost every manufacturer has a type of texture toy on the market. Playskool has a very nice group of three called "Touch 'Ems." Each of these animals—a rabbit, a puppy, and a bear—has seven different textures used on their bodies. These materials are corduroy, satin, felt, ribbing, seersucker, plastic, and cotton. Each of them has bright patterns as well as plain patterns. These give you a lot of opportunity to talk about how these materials feel and to use them to stimulate your baby's sense of touch by rubbing the different textures on his arms, legs, cheek, and stomach. Some words to use when talking about these are:

smooth
soft
rough
bumpy
scratchy
corduroy
satin
felt
ribbed material
seersucker
plastic
cotton

Single Concept

To help your baby understand the meaning of the word "soft," you could say:
Jodie, feel the rabbit's ears. They're sooo *soft*. Doesn't that feel nice? Let's find all the *soft* things. Is the rabbit's arm *soft?* Yes, the arm is *soft*...and a little bit bumpy, too.

Repeat this exercise, placing your child's hand or cheek on each part of the toy animal. Identify all the soft fabrics. You can repeat this at a different time to teach the concept *rough*. Again, go over each part of the textured animal, labeling each part that is rough.
It is best to teach two different concepts, like "soft" and "rough" at different times so your child will not confuse the two.

Don't be afraid to use the actual names of the fabrics when introducing the various textures to your child. Remember, he needs to acquire language receptively before he can expressively communicate back to you. When you label the corduroy "rough" as opposed to the satin "soft," your child gains an understanding of these words as he feels the textures. This kind of sensory impression will help him understand the concept and remember it the next time you use the words "rough" and "soft."

Homemade Toy

Texture Blanket

For a homemade toy for this age group, we suggest that you make a texture blanket. Often we put a blanket down for our baby to lie on to protect him from dirt, dog hairs, or small particles embedded in the carpet. You can protect him with your homemade texture blanket and stimulate him at the same time. If you don't know how to sew or don't have a machine, why not suggest this to one of your friends to make for you as a gift?

To make this blanket, visit the local fabric store and look for their remnant basket. You can make this blanket any size you want and you can use any fabrics that are available there. We suggest that you not use wool for this project. Although the texture of wool is wonderful, there is the possibility that your infant could be allergic to it. Also, you will want to be able to wash the blanket frequently and you cannot always wash wool. Look through this basket of remnants and choose a variety of different textures. You should only need one-fourth to one-half yard of each fabric you want to use. Then take your materials home, wash each of the fabrics, cut them to the shapes that you want, and sew them together. You will enjoy putting your baby on this blanket and allowing him to experience each of these textures. When you have playing time, lie down with him and talk about each of these different materials that you have used. What a treasure for you to keep for your infant to have as he gets older and can understand that this was made just for him.

> ...Oh, would you like to lie down on this nice blanket? Look over here. This is a nice soft blue piece of fabric. (Take his hand.) Can you feel how soft it is? It feels so nice and furry. Oooh, soft! Look at this red part over here. This is corduroy and it feels bumpy. Can you feel how bumpy it is?...

Continue with each of the textures that appear on the blanket. Choose words that accurately describe the feel of the material.

Plate Designs

A simple paper plate can be a fascinating and stimulating toy for your baby at this very young age. Take a plain white paper plate and draw black and white designs on it. If drawing is not for you, then cut pictures or designs from newspapers (black and white) or magazines (color). You may also want to use these to paste some pictures of faces on. Remember that babies of this age enjoy looking at different faces. You can just put the plates in the crib with your child or you can make a mobile with them.

To make the mobile, take a wide piece of ribbon to tie tightly across the side rails of the crib or playpen. Attach another ribbon to the paper plates and then tie this to the wide piece of ribbon. You may want to hang two or three of these at a time. They can be changed as frequently as you wish.

> ...Look, I made you some new designs to look at. Can you see the black lines on this plate? They go swirl, swirl, swirl around and around. Where is the plate? Can you find it? Good! You are looking at the plate....

If you put faces on the plates, you can talk about the facial features as we have shown you before.

> ...Here's a woman. She is looking at you. Do you see her eyes? Her eyes are brown just like yours. Look at her nose. Sniff, sniff. What do you think she is smelling? Maybe she smells her dinner cooking....

Three To Six Months

By the time your infant is three months old, you may be into an established routine. You will be feeling better after the adjustment in your schedule. You will have longer periods of sleep at night, and in fact, your infant may be sleeping through the night during this time period.

She will be more alert and interested in playing with you during these three months of her early life than when she was a newborn. You can continue with some of the activities that we have already talked about and add the new ideas in this section.

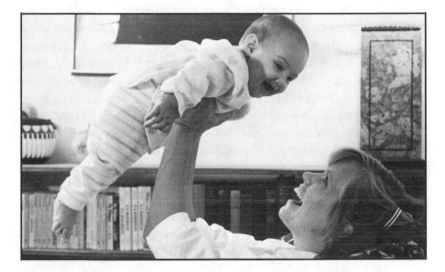

Although your baby may not be quite ready to imitate *you* at this time, it is fun to imitate *her*. If she starts cooing, try to say back exactly what she says. You may be surprised to see that she'll wait for you to make your silly sound and then she'll make hers. This is the very beginning of imitation and is a fun way to spend "diaper changing time." It is also a good way to teach language since imitation is the way that we learn language. Therefore, the more that you and your child can play these babbling imitating games, the more practice she will have making the sounds of our language.

It's important that she have time alone to play around with all of these sound combinations. It is also important that she have you around some of the time to reinforce those sounds and to play babbling games with her. When you reinforce her "talking" she learns that she is communicating with you. It's up to you to provide the correct model for the word that she is saying. If you imitate back to her, she will enjoy beginning to play an imitating game with you. It is a good idea for you to reinforce her accidental combinations of sounds that sound like real words. This gives her a sense of competence in communicating something to you. Remember she really doesn't know exactly what she is saying nor does she attach real meaning to your words.

Let's look at an example of how your reinforcement of her accidental combinations of sounds might happen. She's babbling away and accidentally latches onto the vocal combination of "mamamamama." You will want to jump right in with "You're right little one, here's mama. Mama. I'm your mama." She may look at you quizzically and respond back with "tata." But rest assured, you have done your part. Each time she gets reinforced for saying a new combination that is meaningful, you will encourage her to vocalize more and more. She is just playing with sounds but she is aware when she's listening to what you are saying.

Mobiles

You may want to talk to a friend who has a baby the same age as yours and talk about sharing mobiles. By this time you and your baby have looked at and talked about the same mobile for three months. You both are probably pretty bored with it and it has become something that is just hanging there. If, however, you and your friend have different mobiles, now would be a good time to exchange them. This will give you both a boost.

The mobile that we suggest for this age is the voice-activated one that is made by Johnson and Johnson. It turns on with voice and turns off when the vocalizing stops. Your infant will be cooing and vocalizing more and more during these months and she can learn that she can control a part of her environment by talking. There is no greater motivation for talking than seeing the results of your actions. This mobile is turned on by sound. Your baby can lie in her crib and coo and babble and see the effect on this mobile. You can show her how this works by demonstrating with your own babbling and showing her how it stops and starts depending on whether you are using your voice or not.

> ...Look at the mobile. It is going round and round. Shh, I'll be quiet now. (Whisper.) It stopped moving now. Watch! Mmmmm. See how it moves around? Can you make that sound?...

Your child will not be imitating you at this point yet, but encouraging her vocalizations and having her see that she can control her environment in this way is a good beginning to imitation games.

Special Considerations

If you have found by now that your child has a hearing impairment, you will want her to be able to "see" the results of her vocalizations to supplement whatever she is hearing through her hearing aids. If she has a physical disability and doesn't have much control over her arms or legs, she will feel control by being able to activate this toy by her voice. In fact, if she may need to use voice–activated equipment in the future, this is an excellent start for her. For a number of reasons, this is an excellent toy with which you can interact with your baby.

Mirror

There is really no special age category for this wonderful and unique learning toy. You can put a mirror into your baby's crib on the day that you bring her home from the hospital. We are not sure exactly how much she understands of what she sees in those first few weeks but we do know how much she likes to focus on faces and what better face than her own! During this three-month period, you can use the mirror to develop some receptive language for your baby about herself. Looking in the mirror and pointing out her body parts is a lot of fun.

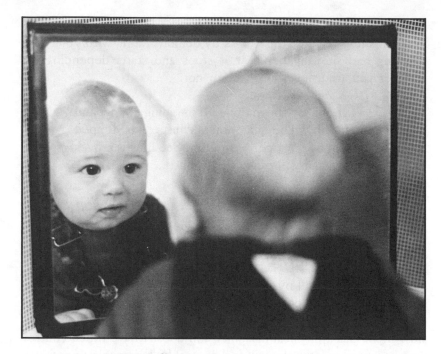

> ..Hi there, Jill. Look at you there in the mir-
> ror. I can see your nose. Yup, right there. Where
> are your eyes? Those are your eyes...

Continue in that way, pointing out all of the baby's body parts and watch her giggle with glee as she watches you touching her body and sees the same thing happening in the mirror. It is your baby's first mystery! How does this happen to me and that baby in the mirror?

The mirror also helps your baby to see herself as separate from you. Early on infants do not know that they are separate from the people around them. This is something they need to learn. As you play with the mirror, she can begin to see that there are two separate people there. One of those people is touching her and *she* is the other one. It is an interesting thing to think about when you're play-ing with her in this way.

Introducing your baby to body parts early helps her develop a self-identity—an identity apart from you—as well as labeling that vocabulary for her. Almost every test of early infant cognitive abilities has sections which test whether she knows where her body parts are. These are part of the development of intellectual skills.

A mirror is a wonderful toy to have. Many of the infant toy manufacturers make one. We will caution you to make sure that the one that you purchase is made of an unbreakable material and provides an accurate reflection. Some have a very distorted image and you would want to check that out before you buy it. Another nice feature of many baby mirrors is that they can be attached to the crib or playpen. A free standing mirror might be hazardous if your infant were to reach out and knock it down on herself. Check for these features before you buy.

Play Gym

A play gym provides a variety of sensory stimulation for your infant and gives you interesting things to talk about as you interact with this toy. A word of caution first. As long as you are with your baby and this toy, there is nothing to worry about, but as she approaches five to six months and can pull the toy with more strength, you will want to remove it from her crib or playpen when you are not with her. Because it is strung across the crib rails she could easily get tangled up in it if she is very agile.

The Fisher-Price Play Gym has a roll-around rattle ball with colored beads, a spinning disk, a bar to grip onto, and sliding daisies. The toy is brightly colored and we encourage you to talk about the colors of each of the objects. All of the spinning and rolling activities encourage focusing on objects. Your infant should be able to do this for increasingly longer periods of time, particularly toward the end of this time period. The bar which she can grip onto is an infant sized version of a chin-up bar. You will want to help her grip this and pull herself up. Do not leave her unattended to do this because in the first part of this time period she will not be able to let go herself and may get "hung-up." Encourage her to reach out to these objects and help her do the actions involved.

Single Concept

Here's the rattle. Can you feel how *round* it is? It goes *round* and *round*, *round* and *round*. You make it go *round* and *round*. There you go—good job. You made it go *round* and *round*. Listen to the sounds that it makes when it goes *round* and *round*. Those sounds are from the little beads inside. They are very small. *Round* and *round*. Good for you. Can you find the spinning disks now?

Again, notice that we keep our sentences short and focused on the item that we are talking about. Remember that in these beginning ages she takes in ideas and vocabulary, but is not ready to give back anything. We must build her receptive language so she will have language concepts to use when she is ready. This is especially true for a child who has a language delay.

Special Considerations

If your child is visually impaired, she will enjoy this activity more if you put the play gym close within her reach, guide her hands to the different objects, and describe them in detail to her.

Doll

Dolls are the toys that are most associated with childhood. Dolls today are available with different complexions so that all children can identify with them. We can use dolls to help our children in many ways. We can bathe dolls and use them to calm fears our babies may have about getting their hair wet or their faces wet.

...My, how Dolly likes to have her face washed.
The water must feel cool and gentle...

We can feed dolls and introduce new foods to our baby through them.

...See Dolly open her mouth. She is going to
try the smooth green peas. Yummy! Dolly likes
peas...

We can use dolls to introduce hospital procedures that may have
to be performed on our own little child. Your child can use her doll
to act out fears and feelings that she is unable to express any other
way.

...Today's the day you're going to see Dr. S.
for your check-up. I'll be Dr. S. and Dolly will be
you. First I'll look at your eyes. Mmm, they look
pretty and blue. Now I'll check your ears. No
problem there...

During these months we suggest you use a doll that has no features that can come off. Everything is sewn onto the soft body.
There are several different dolls made by different manufacturers
but all are very similar. The doll looks human but is soft and stuffed
like a stuffed animal. It can be mouthed and explored without worry
about any loose parts coming off and injuring your baby. Because
it is made of cloth, it is easy to wash and keep clean. This doll can
be used for talking about body parts and facial features just as we
used the stuffed animal in the age grouping of newborn to three
months. Let's use a bedtime scene to illustrate the use of this doll
as a teaching technique for behaviors we want our baby to follow.
It seems that this night is one that your baby has decided to be
fussy about going off to sleep. We get our doll and have a conversation like this:

...Well, it's time to go to sleep now. Dolly is
tired and wants to go to sleep. (Yawn). Wow, Dolly
is really sleepy. Did you see her yawn? Let's put
Dolly to sleep now. She can sleep right in here with
you. You need to be quiet now so that Dolly can
go to sleep. Shhhhhh. Good night now...

You can use this doll when you are playing with a mirror as well. She can be another person whose facial features and body parts can be compared. You can do exercises with the doll that may be ones that your baby needs to do every day and may find uncomfortable. You can show your baby how we do these exercises on the doll. This becomes an especially valuable tool as your child gets older and perhaps resistant to some of the things she will need to do for her therapy sessions. We have often used dolls in language lessons who "talk" for the child. Have the doll join you in your babbling games as you imitate and babble with your infant. Putting the doll in front of your face gives your baby something to focus on while you do the babbling from behind the doll. This also gives your infant an opportunity to listen carefully, since your face is not visible to her.

We're sure that you will think of many other ways that you can play with a doll. Until your child is older, you will want to resist getting the dolls that wet, cry, eat, and do all sorts of other things. Your baby is not ready for so sophisticated a doll and it will not fill any need for her at this time.

Homemade Toys

A Book About Faces

The homemade toy we suggest for this developmental age is a loose-leaf notebook and some 8x10 picture album inserts. Cut out pictures of people's faces from magazines. Find as many different kinds of people as you can. Remember, infants are intrigued by looking at faces. They are more interested in this than just about any other activity. These photo album pages can be removed one at a time and placed in the infant's crib so that she can look at them during her periods of quiet between sleep, playing, or feeding. If you have them between plastic, then she can reach out and touch them but not tear them or get pieces of paper in her mouth. When you talk to her about the pictures, you choose a new and different face each time. You will still be talking about facial features but she will be seeing the same features in various faces. She is learning about worlds beyond her very own although she certainly is not aware of this at this time. Later, when she is old enough to handle

the information, you can talk about different aspects of these people
as you go through her picture book.

>...Here's a picture of a baby girl. She looks like
>you. Here's her eyes. Look at her mouth. It's just
>like your mouth...

Point to your child's features as you talk about the faces.

When your child is older, perhaps between one and two years
of age, you can use this notebook again in a different way. You can
turn it into a vocabulary book.

>...Let's look at this magazine. Can you find a
>picture of *pants?* Good! You found some pants. Do
>they look like your pants? Yes, they have small
>bears just like your pants do. Let's cut out those
>pants and paste them in your book. Can we find
>pants like Daddy wears? Here are some. These are
>blue like Daddy's pants. See how long the legs are.
>Daddy's pants have long legs. Your pants have short
>legs...

Continue as long as your child is interested or until you've filled
the page. Print the word *pants* at the top or bottom of the page.
Now you have started a vocabulary book.

This loose-leaf notebook will be used again and again as your
child grows. As parents, we used this kind of vocabulary notebook.
Together, we and our children looked through magazines for toys,
clothing, and foods that our children could identify. By pasting these
into our first "reader" our children could "read" the pictures to us.
As your child's vocabulary and language grows, you can add sentences to your pictures. You can put in souvenirs of experiences they
have had. Perhaps that first trip to McDonald's could be recorded
with the wrapper from the french fries or a napkin showing those
golden arches. This book for our children became a prized posses-
sion as they "read" it to other family members who visited. If Mom
or Dad is away on a business trip, your child can fill you in with
her activities while you were away by "reading" her book to you.

We do not suggest that all of these are activities that you will want to do at *this* age level but you can start this notebook now for her with pictures of faces and then add to it as she is ready.

Holiday The Year Round

You can make a wonderful visual stimulation toy for your child at this age from the blinking lights that can be found during the holiday season. These lights are inexpensive and you only need a few. Buy a string with blinking lights of different colors. Sew them to a piece of felt. Attach the felt to a dowel and hang on the wall across from her crib, over the changing table, or near her playpen. A very important word of caution here. These are electric lights. They must be plugged in. As with all other electric things, **DO NOT LEAVE YOUR INFANT UNATTENDED** where she can reach the outlets or the lights. Make sure that the plugs and outlets are well out of her reach.

You will have an opportunity to talk about the following ideas:

1. The lights blinking on and off.

2. The colors of the lights.

> ...Look at the pretty lights. They're blinking on and off, on and off. Now they're on. Now they're off. This one is red—now it's off; now on—off—on. Do you see the yellow one? It goes on and off too...

Six To Nine Months

At this developmental age, your baby is able to do more and more things that he could not do before. If he has no physical limita-

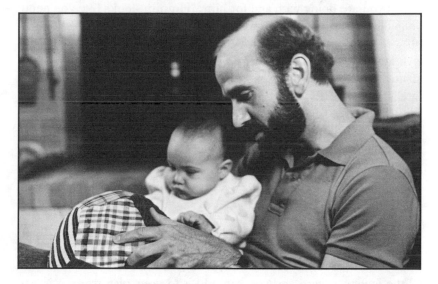

tions, he will be able to sit alone for long periods of time, which will give him a whole new perspective on the world and also make it easier for him to play with you. He is able to pick up and hold objects, which will allow him to be more involved in playing with you. You will begin to see more play that involves both of you in the activity, including times when he will initiate the fun.

During this age span, your baby should be able to sit in a high chair comfortably. If he has physical limitations, he may be able to sit in a specially constructed chair with support.

A word is in order here for "baby talk." It is our opinion that baby talk on the part of the baby is cute but on the part of the parents, unnecessary. It is cute when a one-year-old asks for his "baba" but when the same child does this at age five, it is less appealing. When he asks for his "baba," we can respond with, "Sure I'll get your bottle." We have told him that we understand his communication but this is what it really sounds like. This way you will have less correcting to do when he is older.

While he is beginning to communicate with you by crying and cooing, keep in mind that he is also on the receiving end of the communication. Talk to him about your everyday activities and things you are doing with and for him. "Hmmm, looks like you need your diaper changed. Shall we go and get you a clean one? Okay, off we go." Remember receptive language must come *before* expressive language. He'll enjoy hearing your voice and begin to understand what you are saying months before he will be able to say any intelligible words.

If he has a sensory deficit, he will also learn from the tone of your voice and the way in which he is handled and touched. These added clues are important to the way in which he will learn language.

Rings On A Cone

This toy has many different play possibilities. We will talk about five different concepts you can teach with this toy. You will not want to talk about all of them at this age. However, we'll give you all the language here and you can add it to your play when it is appropriate for your child.

Motion Concepts

Your child will be interested in pulling the rings off before he is physically able to put them back on.

> ...All right, Danny, let's take the rings. Can you pull it off? Pull. Pull. Good for you! You pulled the purple one off. Can you give the purple one to me? Thank you. Let's pull the next one off. That one is yellow. Pull it off. Pull. O.K. Now we pulled off two rings....

Continue until you have them all in your lap. Because he doesn't know the sizes yet, you can hand him the appropriate sizes in order to put the rings back on. Then give him the language for this activity.

> ...Put the red ring on. Do you need some help?
> Put it on. Good! You put it on....

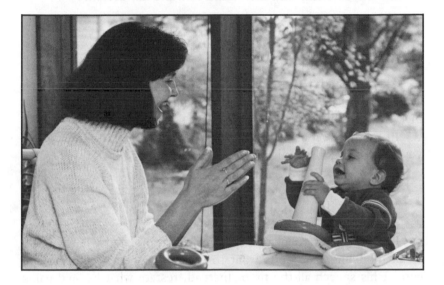

Continue until all the rings are back in place.

Color Concepts

In these early months, talking about the colors will be only an introduction to them for your baby. He probably will not understand all the color words. However, we encourage you to use the color names because, as we have said before, he will need to hear thousands of repetitions before he understands or uses those words.

> ...Look at all the pretty colors on this toy—red,
> green, yellow, orange, blue, purple. This ring is red.
> Here's a green ring. This one is blue....

At this age, you are naming colors, but later on you might want to see if your child can choose between colors which would show his understanding of the words. To play this way, you would put all the rings in your lap. Then take two different colors, and put them in front of your child and say, "Which is the red ring? Can you find the red one? Good for you—you picked the red ring."

If your child chooses the wrong color, tell him the correct name for the one he chose and then hand him the correct one.

> ...That color is blue. Here is the red ring. Can
> you give the red ring to me? Good job....

As your child begins to understand the colors, you can add one at a time until he has all the colored rings in front of him and can pick the one that you ask for.

In another year or two, when he can say the names of the colors, your play can go like this.

> ...What color is this ring? Can you tell me the
> name? That's right—it's red....

If your child's articulation is not clear, remember what we said about modeling. You don't want to become a speech clinician and correct his speech all the time. Instead, restate what he said using the correct pronunciation.

Size Concepts

As with colors, your child is not ready to learn size differences now. However, at a later time, you can use this toy to teach size differences because the rings are graduated from large to small. You would do this in the same way as you did with the colors. The difference is that the colors are distinct from each other but the size is only relative to the next size. We suggest you save this concept until he is two or three years old. Here are some ideas for introducing size concepts.

> ...Let's take off the smallest ring first. The
> smallest ring is purple. The next ring is a little big-
> ger....

Compare the two to see that one is a little bigger. Continue in this way, comparing each ring to the next larger size. When you put them back on, you'll be comparing smaller and smaller sizes. Eventually you should be able to have all the rings in front of your child and have him put them back on from largest to smallest.

Single Concept

This is the simplest activity to do with the cones.

Look at this new toy that we have to play with. Watch it *rock* back and forth. Can you *rock* it? Good! You can *rock* it back and forth. *Rocking, rocking, rocking.*

Continue taking turns rocking the cones until you see that your child has had enough of this activity.

Soft Blocks

Blocks are also very versatile toys, and your baby can enjoy block play at different levels for many years. He can begin playing with them now and continue into his early school years, when he will build elaborate roads and structures which will be the basis of a lot of his imaginative play for many years.

At this developmental age, your baby will be able to stack two or three blocks on top of each other. You will be able to teach the concepts of *up* and *down* with this toy and we give you examples of dialogues for each concept. We suggest that your first set of blocks be the ones made by Dolly Toy Company called "Sof-Pla Blocks," although others are also fine. The ones we use have the Sesame Street characters on them and give you a chance to talk about these characters as well. Take out the blocks and give your baby a chance to mouth and explore them. Since they are soft and washable this is not a problem.

Single Concept

Now for introducing the concept of *up*. Take the blocks and show him how you can stack one on top of the other.

Here's one block. Now I can put one *up* on top. See it go *up* on top. Here's another one—*up* it goes. Can we do one more? *Up-up-up-up* on top. See, we made the block go *up*.

This toy also lends itself to teaching the concept *down*. We suggest that you try this at a different play session so your child will not be confused by the two concepts.

Single Concept

Do you want to make the blocks fall *down?* It's fun when they all crash *down* to the ground. First let's make a tall tower. Let's make it as high as we can. Great! Now, let's knock it *down*.

Gently take your child's hand and knock down the tower.

Here they come down. Wow, they all fell down.

As you stack the blocks, you can take the new one, start at the bottom of the stack and say "up-up-up" as you pass each block that you have already put down.

The most exciting part of this game for your baby is when they all tumble down. He thinks that is great fun and you will be able to hear him chortling with glee. This kind of fun will carry over into when he builds his own structures and watches them tumble down when the final block is too much. Instead of being upset, he will remember from his infant days with you that tumbling down is half of the fun.

...Here's a block with Ernie on it. Watch Ernie go up on top of Grover. Where's Big Bird? Here he is. Let's put Big Bird on top of Ernie. Uh Oh, Big

Bird's going to make them all tumble down. Where's Grover? Did he get crushed? We can do it again. Up they go....

Stacking Cubes

The stacking cubes are based on the same idea as blocks. You can build them up and knock them down, but they can also be stacked inside of each other. This teaches the concept of size order to things just as the stacking rings does. Later on, this toy is also useful for other activities in the sandbox or in the tub, including filling and dumping. Additionally, many of the stacking cubes available have pictures of animals, such as a horse, cow, or duck on the sides or letters on the bottoms so that you can talk about those things as well.

The stacking cubes fit carefully on top of each other. If your baby has the coordination, he can place them so that they will not

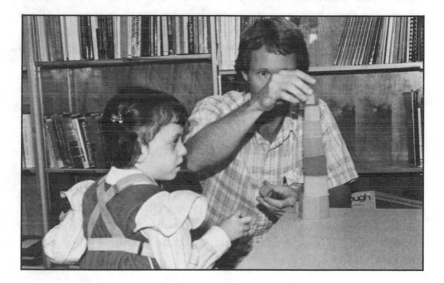

topple over easily. At this developmental age, you will need to help him stack them. Again, your language input will be similar to that used with the blocks and the stacking rings.

> ...These are stacking cubes. Can you take that
> wee small one out? It is very tiny. Can you get it?
> Let me help you. Take it out. There! You did it!
> You took it out. Can you give it to me? Thank you.
> I'll hold them for you over here until we get them
> all out. Let's see about the next one. Here you go.
> Take it out....

Continue in this way until they are all out and then you can help him in the same way to put them back in.

The first skill you should teach with this toy is to take them out of each other with the smallest one first. You will talk about the color of each cube as you take it out and then put it into your lap or on the floor out of sight. When you have them all out, you will want to give him the biggest one and then proceed to stack them on top of each other. You can use the same language as before of "up-up-up," or you can switch to "put it on top," or you can use them both interchangeably. Talk about the colors of the cubes, which are the same primary ones that are used in most of these early toys. You can talk about the pictures that may be on the sides or the bottoms of the cubes. Once you have them all stacked up, you can again say "ooooooh down they go" which is lots of fun.

> ...This cube is the biggest one. We want to put
> it on the bottom. We are building the cubes up.
> Now we put this cube on top of this one. Can you
> put this one on top? Here we go. We are putting it
> on top....

Let's say that you decide during one play session to use the stacking cubes specifically to teach the concept of how things are ordered—in this case from the biggest cube on the bottom to the smallest cube on the top.

Single Concept

Can you find the *biggest* cube?
Motion with your hands spread far apart and say "big" in an exaggerated way.

Yes, there it is. Let's put the *biggest* one right here in front of you. Now, which is the biggest?
Again, use your hands to demonstrate the concept of *big*. Continue this process until you're left with no cubes. Once you have finished stacking all the blocks in order from biggest on the bottom to smallest on the top, go over it again with your child. Look what we did. We put your blocks in order from the *biggest to the smallest*.

The new activity that you can do with the stacking cubes is fitting them inside of one another. At first you will control the actual ordering of the sizes by choosing the block that you give to him. He will not be able to do this himself at this age. You will need to hand him the big one first and then the successively smaller sizes until they are all put back together again. You might want to introduce the idea that there are choices here by saying to your child and yourself as you ponder the cubes:

...Let's see, I wonder which one goes in next? This is a big cube. Now this cube is bigger. Does this cube go inside the other one? Is the rèd one bigger than the blue one? Yes it is. I see. The blue one goes inside the red one....

You might also want to make a "mistake" once in a while and try to fit a larger one into a smaller one and "discover" that it just doesn't work out that way. This little technique will help your baby know that it's okay to make mistakes and that he can't always know the right way to do it.

Balls

Balls are delightful toys and can be used in so many ways and at so many ages. In this section we describe one type that seems just right for this age.

Panosh Place Learning Curves has a "Curiosity Ball." This wonderful toy is soft and round. It can be rolled and tossed and thrown by you and your baby. You can talk about these actions with your baby.

> ...Roll the ball. Good job. Now I'll roll it back to you. I'll roll the ball. Can you crawl over and get it? Great! Bring it back to me now. Can you throw me the ball? Hey, good throw. I can throw it back to you. Oops, you missed. Can you go and get it?...

Besides being "just a ball," this particular toy also unfolds into a play chain of activities. There is a clown face that squeaks and a kitten that fits into a pocket to play "peek-a-boo" with. The kitten has two sides; one side is a sleeping kitten and the other side is an awake kitten. In another section is a small mirror and in another a small rattle. All of these toys can be used to play some of the language stimulating activities that we have already discussed. It is a fun toy to take apart, put back together, or just use as a ball. You can talk about the parts as you unfold it so that you add an air of excitement and mystery to the process.

> ...What's inside? I wonder what we'll find? Oh look! Here's a clown. Do you see the funny clown? Look, there is his big nose. Do you remember where your nose is? Yes, right there....

Continue discussing all of the features and colors of the clown in a similar manner.

The sleepy and awake kitten gives you some new concepts to talk about. Relate these concepts to your baby.

...The little kitten is sleepy. At night you get sleepy, too. Then you go to bed. Shall we put kitten to bed?...

Put him back into his pouch and then pretend that you are sleeping. You might make a noise and say:

...Uh oh, do you think we woke the kitten up? Let's look and see. (Take the kitten out awake side facing your baby.)
Yup—we sure did wake kitten up. You can see kitten's eyes. His eyes are open. So kitten is awake....

The mirror and rattles are additional ways to play with the language that we have already talked about. This toy is very versatile and lots of fun.

Vinyl Books

Your baby has probably just mastered sitting up and you may have begun bathing him in the bathtub. A favorite of many parents is to bathe their infants in the kitchen sink at this in-between stage of being too big for a baby tub and too little for a bathtub. Wherever you bathe him, bath time is now becoming more of an opportunity for play and learning. Your infant is definitely out of that newborn stage where you must be extra vigilant about keeping his body warm. He can now handle changes in body and air temperature and has begun expressing his great pleasure in his bath time.

You will definitely want to keep a firm hold on your baby when you bathe him and for this reason a second adult or older sibling may need to be included.

Because we feel books should be such a large part of your child's language learning, we recommend taking them into the bath as well. This can be done with the soft vinyl, washable books designed specifically for bath time play.

One of the best books for this activity is called *Ernie's Bath Book* (Random House/CTW, 1982). Other alternatives are *Wet Willy's*

Water Fun (Johnson and Johnson), and bath books such as *Freddy Frog*, or *Danny Duck* (Derrydale Books). Each of these books is lightweight and can be fully immersed in the water. These books are particularly useful because they can help provide the basis of your toy dialogues as you study the pictures together.

> ...Ernie's in the bathtub. Ernie's taking a bath just like you, Jason. Can you find Ernie's yellow duck? Where's Jason's duck? Look, Ernie has some soap. Let's find your soap. Now it's time to wash, just like Ernie. See the soap bubbles. They are round. Let's try to pop them...POP!...

Once the washing part of the bath is over, use a few more minutes to explore the sensations of the water. A great deal of language can be drawn from this. Again, refer to Ernie in the book to give your child a clear, visual example of what you are saying.

> ...Ernie's splashing in the water. Now you can splash. (Take your child's hands, and then his feet, and help him splash.) Can you kick your feet, just like Ernie? (Help him kick.) You can pretend to go swimming in the water. (Lightly guide your child back and forth in the tub.)...

Special Considerations

If your child is visually impaired he will be unable to follow along with the pictures in the book. This does not mean you should not read to him. Read the book as you ordinarily would. In this case, since there is little written text, it will be up to you to describe the pictures in clear detail. Describe the characters you see, their size, their color, and their activities. Describe their emotions to your child. Through listening, he will get almost as clear a picture as if he were seeing it himself.

For a language delayed child with a hearing impairment, books in the bathtub—or any time—are wonderful language developing tools because your hearing impaired child will need to rely on his vision. In the bath his hearing aids will be off, so make sure you get good eye contact. Have your child watch your mouth and your facial expressions.

Homemade Toys

Sock Doll

The homemade toy we suggest is a sock doll. This project is very easy to do and requires very little time to make. Take an old, white sock and stuff it with torn nylons or fiberfill. Any material that is washable will do. About one-third of the way down from the toe, stitch around the sock and pull tightly to make the head area. Sew the bottom of the sock doll, which is actually the calf part of the sock, together to close it off. Using different colored threads, sew the features onto the head part of the sock doll. You can even make one side of the doll be an "awake" face and the other side be a "sleeping" face just like the kitten in the "Curiosity Ball." If you feel that your baby has the attention span, you can even make this with him watching. These dolls are soft and cuddly and often become objects that your child will carry around with him for years and years.

Fetch It Toys

Your baby is beginning to understand how to use "tools" to help him reach something. He is beginning to understand cause and effect.

Take a string and tie a toy onto the end of it. Show your baby that if you pull the string the toy will come to you.

> ...I want to get the rattle. The rattle is too far. Oh, I see! If I pull this string, the rattle will come to me. Can you try that? Pull the string and you can get the rattle. Great! You pulled on the string and got the rattle. Good for you!...

In a similar experience, show your baby how to use a stick to bring a toy closer to himself. Put a small toy just out of reach and then use a stick to reach it.

...Watch, I'm going to make the block come to me. See! I can reach out with this stick and poke the block. Poke. Poke. Now see the block is moving toward me. Can you get the block? Use the stick and poke the block. See how it can move to you. You did it!...

Nine To Twelve Months

If this is your first child, you will be astonished at how active your baby becomes in this last part of her first year. You will look back in amazement at all that she has learned. You should also be pleased at how interested she is in playing with you. Her attention

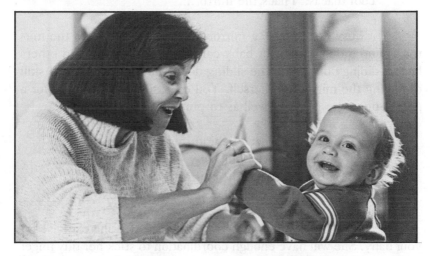

span is longer and she understands more and more of what you say to her. If she has started to walk, she will be running more than she will be walking.

If she has a visual impairment, she may not be as comfortable in another house as she is in yours. Don't hover over her but help her adjust in this new environment. If she has never been there before, you can take her on a tour of the place and tell her where certain things are. For example, "You are standing in front of the couch and there is a small table next to you." Obviously these directions are more than a child of this age will be able to understand, but you are giving her the language at the same time you are giving her a general feel for where things are. She may not understand "small" but "table" will alert her to a possible obstacle. Tell her where you will be and that she can call you if she needs you for any reason.

The toys we suggest in this section are ones that your child will enjoy for many months to come. They include activities that will use many of her new skills and capture her attention.

Playskool Busy Box

There are many variations of this toy. Some go in the crib or playpen, others attach to the stroller or car seat. Choose any one that appeals to you. All of them provide sound and visual stimulation.

> ...Put your hand here. Feel how smooth and cool that is. That's the mirror....

Most busy boxes have a mirror on them. Some have the mirror behind a door that your baby can open and peek at and others have a sliding door. With the sliding door, she can practice the skill of finding the mirror and herself. You can use part of the toy for a peek-a-boo type game as well as to point out facial features.

> ...I wonder what's behind this door. It's a mirror. Who's that beautiful baby in that mirror? Hi, Leah. That's Leah in the mirror. Can you say 'Hi' to yourself? Let's close the door now. Say bye bye now....

The telephone dial on the busy box is a fascinating exercise for your baby. She will have enough coordination to stick her tiny finger through the hole. She may have trouble turning it around all the way but this is where you come in. You can take a turn and show

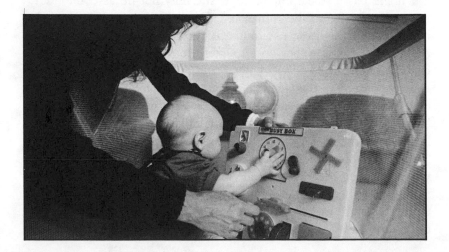

her how it spins and then listen to the clicking noise that it makes as you dial.

> ...Put your finger in that tiny hole. Now you can turn the dial around. Listen. Do you hear that? Click-Click-Click. Watch, I'll show you how. I'm going to put my finger in that tiny little hole and turn the dial. Listen. Click-Click-Click. Do you want to try it now?...

The puppy on this busy box squeaks when it is pushed. Your baby will be able to push by herself and her efforts will be rewarded by that tiny sound.

Single Concept

> Can you *push* the puppy on your busy box? Listen to the tiny sound. (Help your child push on the puppy and signal for her to listen for the sound by putting one of your fingers up to your ears.) I heard it. That's what happens when we *push* the puppy. Did you hear the puppy when you *pushed* him down? Good, you *pushed* the puppy and we heard him. Good job of *pushing* the puppy.

The giraffe rings a bell when the dial is turned. Use action words that go along with the activities. We have named many nouns but we also need to make sure that we teach action verbs. This is a good toy to do that with.

> ...The puppy *squeaks*. The giraffe *rings* the bell. The rabbit *pulls* down. The dial *turns*. The door *slides*. The bees *fly* and another bee *flutters*....

If your baby is up and about, you may want to encourage her to imitate some of these actions. She can fly and flutter like the bees and hop like the rabbit. She may not be perfect at imitating these actions but she will love trying. Don't be embarrassed to join her in this activity. Being a kid again is one of the fun parts of being a parent.

Special Considerations

The sounds that come from a busy box are usually not very powerful and you would not expect your hearing impaired child to be able to respond to them. We suggest that you point out the noises to her and simulate the kind of sound that it makes so that she can hear/see you as well as the toy. Remember to have her focus on your face. Whenever possible, get as close as you can to the toy so that your child can see your face as you are talking while she is still able to look at the toy.

If your child is visually impaired, once again you will want to describe what she is hearing and what the toy looks like. Take her hand and gently guide it over each part of the toy. Carefully describe in detail what each of these objects looks like and how they push, turn, slide, or dial.

Busy Bath

Your baby should be comfortable in the tub at this age and we suggest that you invest in a bath seat with strap so that she can sit without sliding down into the water. *Never* leave your baby unattended in the tub even if she is strapped to a bath seat and even if you will only be gone for a second. Having a bath toy gives you lots of interesting things to talk about and keeps your child involved while you bathe her. It is a good idea to get the business part of the bath done as soon as you put her in. Then when you are finished with the actual bath, you can have play time. You can take her right out when she is tired or loses interest.

As with the other activity toys, there are many fine products on the market today. The one we use is made by Child Guidance and is called "Busy Bath." This toy has a removable cup which you and your baby can fill and spill for as long as she is interested. Some vocabulary that you can introduce for this is:

> ...Fill the cup. It's full. Pour the water. Now it's empty. More—do you want more? That's enough, the cup is full. Pour it on the (wheel, dolphin, water-

go-round, sailboat)....

There is a dolphin on the toy which squirts water. The water pump fills the dolphin with water, then you can squirt the water at the water-go-round which goes around. If you turn the dolphin in the other direction, you can make the water wheel go around and around.

Be sure to use the real words to describe these features. Talk about the "dolphin" and not the "big fishy." Using proper vocabulary at this time saves you from having to go back and teach it again later on.

Remember at this age, your baby is able to imitate some babbling sounds with you and possibly even a few words as she approaches her first birthday. This toy lends itself very well to babbling games.

Use long vowel sounds as you empty the cup: *ee, oo, ah*. Use lip trilling /*brrrr*/ as you make the water wheel and the water-go-round move. Use a "rocking" /*babababa*/ kind of sound as you make the sailboat move back and forth. Your baby will love to play these imitating games.

As we mentioned earlier with the mobiles, you might want to share some of these toys with your friends. There are many types of bath activity boxes, each of which has the same basic kinds of actions on them but different animals and objects do the actions. It will keep the game interesting for your baby if you vary the actual toys that you use. You get double value for your toys this way.

Balls

We have talked about balls before but now that your baby may be up on her feet we can talk about other action words involving balls. A very fine ball to have at this time is a beach ball. It is light, very colorful, and easy for your baby to catch and hold onto because of its size. You can use the beach ball and another ball like a Nerf ball to compare sizes with your baby. Have both balls with you and say to your baby:

...Come and get the big ball. Which is the big beach ball? Good job, you found the big beach ball.

Can you roll it to me? Good work....

Aside from teaching the concept *big,* you can use the balls to teach the concept *round.*

Single Concept

Look, these balls are *round.* (Stress the shape with your hands.) The beach ball is a big, *round* ball. The Nerf ball is a little, *round* ball.

Point out the colors of the balls to your child. Look, your ball is red and yellow. It has stripes on it. Here is a red stripe and here is a yellow stripe.

Statements such as these can help teach your child the concept of colors.

Another concept is that of *action verbs.* You can use these verbs with all the things you can do with a ball.

Single Concept

Can you *roll* the ball to me? I'll *roll* it to you. Let's *roll* it to Henry. Boy, that ball can really *roll.*

Can you *push* the ball? Take two hands and *push* it. *Push* it hard. Great job! You *pushed* it.

Now can you *kick* the ball? *Kick* the ball with your feet. You *kicked* the ball a long way.

Now let's practice *throwing* the ball. Take two hands. Way over your head. Hold onto the ball real tight.... Now, let go. *Throw* it. Great! You did it. You *threw* the ball.

Can you *catch* the ball? Hold out your hands like this. Now you are ready to *catch* the ball. Here it comes. Fantastic! You *caught* the ball.

Now let's *bounce* the ball. *Bounce* it on the ground. Now, *bounce* it high in the air. You can *bounce* the ball very well. Good for you.

Homemade Toys

What's In My Pot?

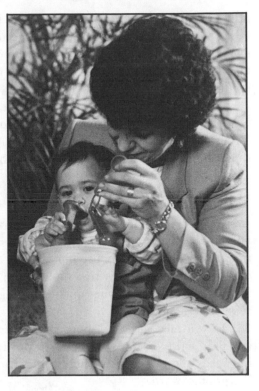

Our homemade toy for this age group can be used for many months to come. You do not actually have to "make" anything. You just need to gather things together. Get several plastic containers such as the ones that ice cream comes in (Well, you don't have to eat it all in one night!) and several types of objects that your baby can put into the containers. Some examples might be: empty film canisters, plastic spoons, plastic measuring spoons, wooden clothespins, and empty spools of thread. Make sure that you do not use very small objects that could be swallowed, sharp objects that could cut, or objects that are breakable. You can talk about each of these kinds of objects as your baby delights in filling and dumping all of these containers. Once again, you can use this toy for a babbling imitation type of game. Hold the plastic spoon up by your mouth and say:

> ...Ooooooooo, down it goes into the bucket. Ahhhhhhhh, here goes another one. Here's one for you. Can you say ahhhhhhhhhhh? Good job of talking! That was great....

Special Considerations

We mentioned earlier that if your baby has a hearing impairment she will need to have many hearing evaluations. She is still a little young to be reliable about using a toy to show us what she hears; however, you can use this game to teach her to wait for a sound and then drop the object into the container when she hears it. With this practice, she can soon be a reliable listener in a hearing test.

If your baby has a visual impairment, you may need to guide her into dropping her objects into the container but don't do this for her for too long. She will be able to judge for herself soon what the relationship of the container to her object is.

Danielle's Story

Do you remember when we talked about picture notebooks, vocabulary books, and experience books? This would be a good time to make a book about your child. Take actual photos of your child doing her daily activities—in her crib; at nap time; eating breakfast; taking a bath; playing outside; going in the car; at a therapy session. Whenever.

As you talk with her about the picture, paste it into the book and then write a sentence about it. We know that she is not reading words yet, but exposing her to print early gets her thinking about the printed word.

> ...Look at this picture, Danielle. This is a picture of you upstairs in your crib. Are you sleepy? There's your rabbit. Time for a nap. Danielle is taking a nap in this picture. Let's paste it in your book. Can you help? I'll put the paste on and you can turn it over. Now let's see—we'll write 'Danielle is taking a nap.' Okay. Let's see Danielle's other pictures....

Continue in this way as long as she stays interested in what you are doing. Add pictures of relatives so that they are available when these people are about to visit. Preparing your child ahead of time allows her time to think about "strange" people coming into her life. If she is going to therapy, be sure to take a picture of her therapist so that on the days when she is going to see her, you can refer to this picture. You can even have a second picture to put up on the calendar on the days when she will be going so that she can see the relation of the calendar to her activity. Again, remember this is at a receptive level. We do not expect her to be at all aware of days of the week at this age.

Summary

Here we are at the end of the first developmental stage. Can you believe how many things your baby is able to do for herself? This is a time of rapid growth and all of the months of building her receptive language will start to pay off. She'll probably be saying one or two words by now and soon this number will increase dramatically.

Vocabulary And Concepts

The following list will give you an idea of the vocabulary and concepts that your child should be familiar with:

action words (push, turn, slide, dial, fly, flutter, fill, pour, roll, kick, throw, catch, bounce, fill, dump)

actions (crawl, walk, jump, run)

alphabet letters

animal names (sheep, horse, kitty, puppy, rabbit, bear)

animal sounds (baa, neigh, meow, ruff)

baby's belongings (cup, bottle, high chair, playpen, crib, spoon)

body and facial parts (eyes, nose, mouth, head, tummy or stomach, arms, legs, fingers, toes)

child's name

clothes (pants, shirt, hat, sweater, shoes, socks, mittens, coat)

colors (black, white, red, green, blue, yellow)

common familiar objects (fruit, toys, foods, instruments, balloon)

daily activities (play in crib or playpen, riding in car, going to the

doctor or therapist, taking a nap, taking a bath)

descriptions of animals (fluffy, has tail, hops)

emotions (happy, sad, laugh, cry)

familiar television characters (Big Bird, Ernie, Bert, Cookie
    Monster)
family member's names
goodbye
hello
lullabies (Hush Little Baby)
materials (corduroy, satin, felt, plastic, cotton)
more animals (cow, duck, fish, squirrel, goat, owl, bird,
    turtle)
more colors (orange, purple)
names of everyday activities (change diaper, bath time, meal-
    time)
numbers 1-10
opposites (up/down, in/out, on/off, back/forth, sleep-
    ing/awake)
round
size discrimination (small, smaller, smallest, big, bigger, big-
    gest)
stripes

Toy Summary

The following is a list of toys that we have worked with in this
first developmental year. The * indicates a homemade toy.

balls	stacking ring
busy bath	*plate designs
busy box	*texture blanket
dolls	*what's in my pot?
mirror	stuffed animals
mobiles	texture toys
picture notebook	*book about faces
play gym	*book about
rattles	my child
sock doll	*containers for
soft blocks	household objects
stacking cubes	*holiday the year round

Books

It is never too early to introduce books at bedtime as a quiet activity before sleep. Usually bedtime is not a problem at this age, but it is a nice ritual to begin.

You will find that your child is much more interested in sitting still for a quiet session of book reading now than when she was younger. She will not be able to follow a complicated story but will enjoy pointing to pictures and perhaps naming a few in some of the early picture books.

ABC An Alphabet Book, Thomas Matthieson, New York: Platt and Munk, 1966.

Photographs of common objects that will be familiar to a young child. A is for apple, B for balloons, G for guitar. The photos are clear with only one to a page. The facing page has the letter and a brief paragraph using the word.

Animal Picture Book, New York: Platt and Munk, 1968.

A board book with large photographic pictures of familiar animals, one to a page. The animals are a squirrel, goats, ducks, rabbit, kitten, owl, puppies, parrot, fish, cat, and turtle. The pictures are labeled with the word. Lots of opportunity here for talking about the animal's features.

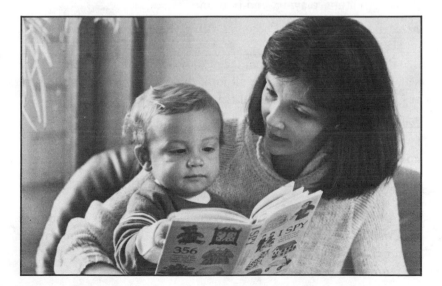

Babies, Gyo Fujikawa, New York: Grossett and Dunlap, 1963.
Board book showing babies being washed, changed, eating, laughing, crying. Babies enjoy seeing pictures of others just like themselves.

Baby's First Cloth Book, George Ford, New York: Random House, 1970.
Cloth book which your baby cannot rip, with pictures of everyday objects.

Baby's First Words, Lars Wile, New York: Random House, 1983.
Board book of photographs of clothes, objects, and actions in a young child's life. Board pages make it easier for baby to turn the pages.

Baby Talk: A Pillow Pal Book, New York: Platt and Munk, 1982.
A soft plastic book that can be chewed, tubbed, and played with. Opens up into one long mural showing pictures of babies at play.

Baby's Things, New York: Platt and Munk, 1978.
Photographs of familiar objects.

Early Words, Richard Scarry, New York: Random House, 1976.
Cardboard pages with little clutter. The objects are easily recognizable. The objects are of daily activities of waking up, washing, dressing, eating, playing, and bedtime.

Faces, Barbara Brenner, Photographs by George Aricona, New York: E.P. Dutton, 1970.
Pictures of many different faces showing features that are all the same but illustrating that we all look different. Introduces the senses that we use with the facial features.

Family, Helen Oxenbury, New York: Wanderer Press, 1981.
This is a board book that talks about members of the immediate and extended family.

Goodnight Moon, Margaret Wise Brown, New York: Harper and Row, 1977.
A classic tale for young children where the little mouse says goodnight to all the objects in her room and also to the moon. An all time favorite with children.

Hush Kitten, Emanuel Schongut, New York: Little Simon Books, 1983.

Two little cats making different sounds, such as crackling leaves, popping balloons, breaking dishes, ripping paper.

I Spy, Lucille Ogle and Tina Thoburn, New York: American Heritage, 1970.

Clear photographs of familiar objects such as toys, food, pets, clothes. A fun book for naming, guessing riddles, and playing "I Spy."

I Hear, Lucille Ogle and Tina Thoburn, New York: American Heritage, 1970.

Same format as the *I Spy* book with these pictures showing sounds that different things make. Some sounds may be out of a young child's realm of experience but the sounds are fun to practice for speech sounds.

Let's Eat, Gyo Fujikawa, Japan: Zokeisha Publications, Ltd., 1975.

Shows children of various nationalities eating different kinds of food—peanut butter and jelly, pizza, a drumstick, an apple, whatever.

My Animal Friends, New York: Grossett and Dunlap, 1981.

A board book with pictures of familiar animals.

My Back Yard, Anna and Harlow Rockwell, New York: Macmillan, 1984.

Shows pictures of objects in the yard such as trees, birds, laundry drying, sprinkler, sandbox, and swing.

My Feet Do, Jean Holzenthaler, Photographs by George Ancona, New York: E.P. Dutton, 1979.

Photographs of a small girl's feet showing left and right, walking, running, jumping, and hopping.

My First Soft Learning Books, New York: Nasta.

These are plastic tub books. One talks about numbers and the other about letters of the alphabet.

My Hands Can, Jean Holzenthaler, Illustrated by Nancy Tafuri, New York: E.P. Dutton, 1978.

Shows the different things that hands can do. They can button, zip, do good things, can hurt, and can show others how we feel.

My Picture Book, New York: Platt and Munk, 1968.

This is a board book showing pictures of cups, spoon, zipper, gloves, house, umbrella, telephone, clock, balls, cookies, pencils. Some of the pictures are a little old-fashioned but they are good for expanding baby's knowledge.

My Shirt Is White, Dick Bruna, New York: Methuen, 1984.

A simple book about color. There is one item of clothing and one color on a page.

My Toys, Dick Bruna, New York: Methuen, 1980.

A board book that folds out to show toys that will be familiar to baby.

Pat The Bunny, Dorothy Kunhardt, New York: Western Publishing Co., Inc.

A hands-on touching book with activities for babies to do, play peek-a-boo, pat the soft cotton on the bunny, look in the mirror, feel daddy's scratchy face, read a small book, put a finger through a ring, and wave bye bye. A long time favorite that will interest young children for many years.

Playing, Helen Oxenbury, New York: Simon and Schuster, 1981.

Simple pictures of babies with different toys such as a block wagon, drums, books, teddy bear, and sitting in a box.

Spot's Toys, Eric Hill, New York: Putnam, 1984.

Vinyl book that can go in the tub with pictures of the little dog, Spot, playing with her toys.

The Me Book, John E. Johnson, New York: Random House, 1979.

A cloth book that names different parts of the body. Baby will enjoy pointing to this own parts as you show them in the book.

The Me I See, Barbara Shook Hazen, Illustrated by Ati Forberg, New York: Abingdon Press, 1978.

In a lovely, rhymed text, parts of the body, senses, and functions of each are shown.

Touch Me Books, P. and E. Witte, Illustrated by H. Rockwell, Wisconsin: Golden Books, 1961.

Different textures such as sponges, wood, furry things on each page.

What Do Babies Do? Debby Slier, New York: Random House, 1985.

A board book with pictures of babies doing everyday activities such as sleeping, eating, looking in a mirror.

What Is It?, Tana Hoban, New York: Greenwillow Press, 1983.

Excellent photographs of everyday objects in a baby's life.

The next few pages are checklists to help you evaluate how your child is progressing.

SUMMARY OF YOUR CHILD'S FIRST YEAR 0-12 MONTHS

LANGUAGE

Developmental Milestones	Date Achieved	NOT YET	PROGRESSING
cries to express needs			
makes vowel-like cooing sounds			
responds by smiling to friendly faces			
turns to sound			
laughs out loud			
vocalizes when spoken to			
uses her voice to express needs			
babbles several consonants			
"talks" to toys			
"talks" to mirror			
responds to name			
stops action when "no" is said			
waves bye bye			
nods head for "yes"			
responds to "yes/no" questions			
enjoys music and rhymes			
one or two words			

PHYSICAL

Developmental Milestones	Date Achieved	NOT YET	PROGRESSING
follows a moving person			
follows a moving object			
focuses on hands			
brings hand to mouth			
can hold on to rattles			
plays with fingers			
plays with hands			
can move object from one hand to another			
can crawl			
can sit alone			
can clap hands			
can drink from a cup			
can roll a ball			
can creep upstairs			
can walk with one hand held			
can walk alone			
moves body to music			
can build a tower of blocks how many?			
can put objects into containers			
can dump objects out of containers			
can pick up small objects			

COGNITIVE

Developmental Milestones	Date Achieved	NOT YET	PROGRESSING
responds to visual stimulation			
responds to touch stimulation			
responds to sound stimulation			
focuses on faces			
discriminates between family and strangers			
enjoys being with people			
raises arms when told "up"			
responds to name			
discriminates between friendly and angry voices			
understands bye bye			
can follow a single direction "come here" "stand up"			
has exposure to colors red green blue yellow black white			
has exposure to facial parts			
has exposure to vocabulary of textures smooth scratchy bumpy rough soft			

Twelve To Fifteen Months

During this developmental period you will begin to see your play with the dialogues pay off. Your toddler understands more and more of what you say. He should be able to go and get an object that you ask him for, such as his ball or doll. He will be able to choose between two colors when you ask him to hand you the red one with only two to choose from. He will be on the go all of his waking hours. Encourage his participation in clean up time. Make this a ritual before bedtime or whenever it is convenient for you. If you join him in the clean up and make it a language learning time, it will be enjoyable for both of you. This is a good time for you to practice his ability to go and get objects that are familiar to him.

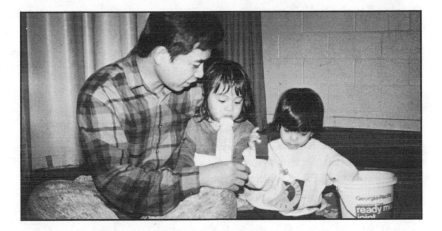

...Bring me the doll. Good! I'll put the doll on the shelf. Now get the big giraffe with the long neck. He goes on the top shelf because his neck is so long. Can you reach the top shelf or shall I lift you up? Ooooo, he's tall and so are you. Up it goes. Now we have all of your nice toys ready to go to sleep and ready to play with you tomorrow. Let's choose our story now....

It is fun to listen to a child of this age with a toy telephone because you will hear him using your tones and your inflections. Once you have realized how easily your child can imitate tones and inflections, you will want to pay attention to how you use your voice with him. Your tone and your inflections carry a lot of meaning for him. He will need to learn to understand your tones of love and caring as well as the tones you use when you disapprove of what he has gotten into. While he is learning to talk, walk, and interact with you, he is also learning about his feelings. You can teach him about his feelings by telling him how you feel at different times. Repeat in meaningful ways how much you love and care for him, your pleasure in him, and your joy in being with him. Communicating feelings of love will help him to grow with confidence and self-esteem.

Push And Pull Toys

This is an active period for your toddler. If he is physically able, he will be up on his feet during this time. He will be able to push toys forward before he will be able to pull them with a string. A fine push toy that most toddlers enjoy is a toy lawn mower. We do not recommend that your youngster follow you along as you mow the lawn because it is too dangerous. However, he can pretend to cut the lawn either before or after you do. There is good language that can be learned from this chore. You can introduce the concepts of "before" and "after" by talking about how tall the grass is before you cut it and how short it is after you cut it. Talk about the need for sun and rain to make the lawn grow. During the week you can talk about the weather and the effect that it might have on the grass. Your toddler will not have a very good grasp of all of this scientific data, but remember you are building receptive language skills all the time and these are always ahead of his expressive skills.

Single Concept

It's time to cut the grass because the grass is too *tall*. What makes the grass grow *tall?* The sun makes the grass grow *tall*. The rain makes the grass grow *tall*. The grass is *tall* before we cut it. Now let's get the lawn mower and cut the grass.

Will the grass be *tall* after we cut it? No. But the sun and rain will help the grass grow *tall* again.

Your toddler can also help you in the house by pushing the vacuum cleaner with you around the living room. You may have to go back later to actually get the job done but he will feel big and important in helping you with this household chore. Once again you can talk about the carpet being dirty before you vacuum and how nice and clean it is after.

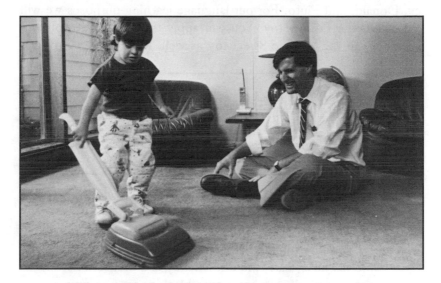

To fully enjoy a pull toy, your child will need to be able to walk forward while looking back to pull a string toy. Many of these toys make clicking or clacking sounds and they are fun to talk about. One toy that he might enjoy is the Playskool Block Wagon. This wagon is small and holds about twenty-four blocks. It has a string on it that he can pull.

...Where is your block wagon? Can you go and get it? Bring it to me so that we can build something with the blocks. That's right—you found it! *Pull* it to me. The wagon is *behind* you when you *pull* it. *Pull* the wagon. Good for you. You *pulled* the wagon over to me....

Surprise Box

This is one of our favorite toys and will stay a favorite with your toddler for a long time. Your language teaching time at this age will be about the names of the objects that are in your surprise box as well as the different actions required to make them pop up.

Playskool makes both a Busy Poppin' Pals which has the Sesame Street characters of Ernie, Bert, Big Bird, Oscar, and Cookie Monster, and Disney Poppin' Pals which has Goofy, Dumbo, Mickey, Donald, and Pluto. For our language learning purposes we will talk about the Disney toy. You can apply the same types of conversations to the Sesame Street toy as well.

Single Concept

Let's name all the *animals* in your surprise box. There's Goofy, Dumbo, Mickey, Donald, and Pluto. So many *animals*. Which *animal* do you like best?

...Goofy is a dog. He has long floppy ears, a big black nose and a mouth. Dumbo is an elephant. He has huge ears. In the circus he learned how to fly. Do you think an elephant can really fly? Show me his nose, ears, mouth. Mickey is a mouse. His ears are black. He has a cute black nose. Can you find his mouth? Donald is a duck. His beak is yellow. When he talks, he says quack, quack, quack. Pluto is another kind of dog. Can you find his nose? Do you know what color his nose is?...

There is a dial under Goofy that turns. Can you turn the dial? Round and Round. POP! There's

Goofy. Under Dumbo is a lever that you can pull
down. Can you pull the lever? POP! There's
Dumbo. Under Mickey is a bar that slides. Watch,
here's how the slide works. POP! There's Mickey.
Under Donald there is a knob that turns. Can you
turn it? Turn it over. POP! There's Donald. Under
Pluto there's a button that you push that also makes
a squeaky noise. Push. POP! There's Pluto....

Single Concept
Where is the dial that turns? You're right! It's
under Goofy. See it *under* Goofy? Can you find
Dumbo? There is a lever *under* Dumbo. Boy, there
sure are a lot of things *under* these animals. Oh, I
see a knob *under* Donald. Is there anything *under*
Pluto? Let's see! You're right. There is a button
under Pluto.

Now that you have introduced all of the actions and some of
the vocabulary concepts, you can play a game with all of the characters. With your toddler watching, you push down the lids of each
character one by one. Say "Bye-bye Mickey, Bye-bye Donald." All
the way down the list of characters. When all of the lids are closed
you can cover all of the lids except one and ask:

...Where is Goofy? Do you know where he is?
Right, he's under this one. Can you wake him up?...

After your toddler turns the dial and Goofy pops up you can
say:

..Hi, Goofy. Were you sleeping? Wake up time.
Now I wonder who's under this next one....

Continue until you have all of the characters up again. In this
way you have repeated the words "hi," "sleeping," and "wake up"
five different times as well as action words and the names of the

characters. That's quite a bit of language for about five minutes of play time.

Once you have all of the characters up, you can proceed one by one to put them back to sleep.

> ...Oh, Donald looks sleepy. Let's tell him bye bye and put him back to sleep. Bye bye, Donald....

If you control each character by covering the others with your hand, you will be encouraging your toddler to wait for your direc-

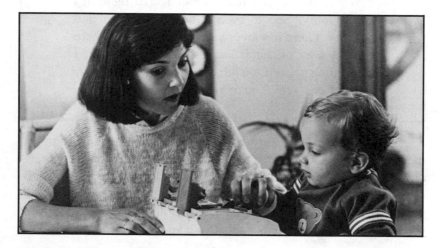

tion and to curb his impulsiveness. He will also be learning to take turns.

There is a tremendous amount of language that you can teach with this simple toy. You'll think of even more fun things to do with it as you go along.

Floating Family Water Toy

This toy is fun for the bath, wading pool, or sink. There are three sturdy objects which are weighted and float nicely: a boat, a cup, and a turtle. There are three men who fit into holes in these objects. A perfect time for the nursery rhyme, "Rub-a-dub-dub—three men in a tub." Of course you will want to name the objects for your toddler. After you have told him the names, you may want to ask him to hand you specific ones.

>...Can you find the turtle? Where is the boat? Can you give me the cup?...

Then you can expand it to include more vocabulary.

>...Which one is the boat? I see a man taking a ride in the boat. He is sailing his boat in the water. Can you push the boat in the water? Good job.
>
>Now, do you see the turtle? He's the little green animal that lives in the water. The turtle likes to float in the water. Just like you. The turtle floats and the boat does too. What a fun toy!
>
>See the cup. You can fill the cup with water. Now you can pour the water out of the cup. And now you can fill the cup again. Good for you. Can the cup float? What happens when you fill the cup with water? Does it float like the turtle?...

Some vocabulary concepts that you can teach with this toy are:

put it in
take it out
give me the
hand me the
show me the
where is the
float the boat (turtle, cup, man).
colors—blue boat, green turtle, blue cup

You will find that this toy will be used for many different activities during its lifetime and will hold up very well.

The toy comes with a cup and you might be tempted to pretend to drink from it. We discourage you from doing this since it implies to your toddler that you can drink the bath water. It might be better to keep drinking activities to feeding time in the kitchen at the table or high chair.

Homemade Toys

Playdough

Another classic toy that you can make easily at home is Playdough. There are many recipes for this mixture. We include two here; one that you can eat and one that you cannot. The one that you should not eat is not toxic; it just is not very tasty.

Nonedible Playdough

1 1/2 cups flour	1/4 cup vegetable oil
1/2 cup salt	liquid food colors
1/2 cup water	

Mix the food color with the water before adding to the flour mixture. The color will be more even this way. You will want to talk about the colors as you decide which color to make the playdough. When your child is four or five, you can talk about how you can mix colors together to make different colors. For example, red and blue mixed together make purple, and blue and yellow mixed together make green.

Mix flour and salt together. Add water and oil and knead the dough well. If you leave your finished product out in the air, it will harden. If you do not want your dough to harden, put it in the refrigerator in a covered jar and it can be used again.

Peanut Butter Playdough

2 cups peanut butter
2 cups powdered milk
1 cup honey

Mix all of the ingredients together. Add more powdered milk to make it less sticky. You can roll and form this playdough the way you did with the first one but you would not want to make too much or keep it too long. Once you have played with it and eaten as much as you both want, put it in the refrigerator to keep it cool.

You can keep your playdough in covered containers for several days in the refrigerator without it spoiling. Making the playdough together with your child is a wonderful time to introduce measuring concepts. He can help you measure, pour, and mix.

> ...Oh, Jamie, it's raining out today and we won't be able to go to the park. I have an idea. Would you like to help me make some playdough? Let's see if we have what we need. Let's look in the cupboard. We need flour. Do you see the flour? Right, there it is. Okay, can you find the salt? Good!
>
> We need salt also. Now where is the oil? Oh, I see it—way in the back. Can you carry the salt? Good! Bring it to the table. Up you go—come on up where you can see and help. I'll measure the flour and you can dump it in the bowl. Good job! We have flour in the bowl. Now we need the salt. I'll measure the salt. Can you dump that in the bowl? Now you can mix it up with this big spoon. Good. Now we're ready to add the liquids. We need water and oil. What color should we make the play-dough? We have red, green, yellow, and blue....

Point to each as you name them. Your child does not know colors at this age. When he points to one, tell him again what color it is.

> ...Okay, you want to make yellow playdough today. Yellow is a good color for today because the sun is not shining and we can still make it a sunshiny day. What a good idea you had. Now we can pour the water into this small bowl. Then we can add the oil. You did that very well. Do you want to squeeze the yellow food color? Oops, that's a lot of yellow in there. Okay, we will have a very bright playdough. Now we can add the liquid to the flour and then mix up our playdough....

This may be the end of your child's attention for now. If so, put the playdough in a covered container and put it away for now. There is no limit to what you can do with playdough. Most children this age just enjoy the squooshing and squeezing of the material. Do not interfere with this, but you can have your own plan in mind of what you are going to make with yours. We have always had fun making balls out of the playdough and rolling them across the table to the child to roll back to us. Another favorite which encourages new language concepts are *loooong* snakes and short snakes which are rolled out. If you want to get fancy you can use a rolling pin and cookie cutters to make different shapes that you can discuss and perhaps even create a story about. Let your imagination run wild with this wonderful, expandable toy.

> ...Jamie, would you like to make something with
> your playdough now? Can you get it from the shelf?
> Here's some for you and I'll play with some....

It's important that you follow your child's lead here and be ready to comment on whatever he's making without making him do what you are doing. Very young children will probably be mostly squeezing and mushing the dough. Comment on what he is doing and then add comments about what you are making.

> ...You like to squeeze the playdough. It feels so
> good when you are squooshing it between your
> fingers. I'm going to roll my playdough. Oh, look.
> I made a long rope. Now I can make a short one.
> This one is long and this one is short. Did you make
> a short rope too? Good work. Let's see what else
> we can make. I made a small ball. Shall I roll the
> ball to you? (This is a great time for an impromptu
> 'roll the ball' game.)...

Anticipate when he is tiring of the activity so that you can leave enough time for him to participate in clean up with you.

At another time, you may want to try different shaped cookie cutters with the playdough. If you have them, you can match your

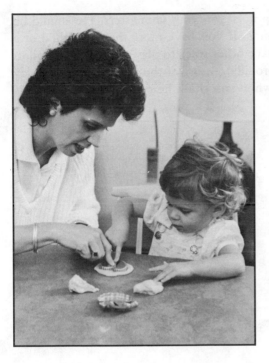

cookie cutters to whatever vocabulary you may want to work on. There are animal cookie cutters, toy cutters, and holiday ones. Many plastic toys can also be used as cookie cutters for playdough since the playdough washes off easily.

Large Boxes

When you watch your child unwrap his gifts at holiday or birthday time, you may have been amused to see that he loved the boxes the gifts came in almost as much as the gifts themselves. We suggest that you have some large boxes around for your toddler to play in, on, under, and anywhere else he can get himself into. Our favorite has always been the boxes that refrigerators come in. You can usually check at a new home construction site and talk with the site manager. He can let you know when they will be delivering the home appliances. Your child will enjoy making his box into a play house, boat, car, airplane, and whatever else his imagination leads him to. Your play with him might be like this.

> ...Do you want to play in your huge box today? What shall we make it? An airplane—okay. Do you want to be the pilot or a passenger? Okay, I will be the passenger then. Wait a minute and let me get my suitcase. (This can be pretend or real.) Okay, I'm ready now. I will sit in my seat and put on my seat belt. Are we ready for take off?...

Encourage revving-up noises in your youngsters. He should be able to imitate these sounds. If you have more than one child or a playmate over, you can have other roles to play such as the co-pilot. At this age you will be providing most of the dialogue for this play but remember to pause when you think he can supply some words to this play.

Fifteen To Eighteen Months

You will notice your active toddler becoming even more active during these few months. She can climb now and you need to be careful of dangerous things, not only on the floor but at any other level as well. There is no place that she cannot get to at this time. Safety first. If you think she can't, she will. She is also walking well by this time. She rarely falls. When she is running, she still may fall because her feet tend to get ahead of her. She will enjoy moving in time to music.

She will also enjoy scribbling with crayons and markers. When buying crayons and markers, get the kind that are rather fat. These are easier for her to hold. At this stage she will be holding the crayons in her fist rather than as you would hold a pencil. That is fine for this developmental age.

You will want to keep these crayons under your control. They often end up being used to decorate walls and furniture. We do not recommend coloring books at this age since your child is only able to scribble and is not able to color within lines. She will be able to color within lines by the time she is five. For now large blank pieces of paper or a roll of white shelving paper is perfect. Be aware that she may go off the paper so you want to make sure the surface that she is coloring on is washable or covered with a layer of newspaper.

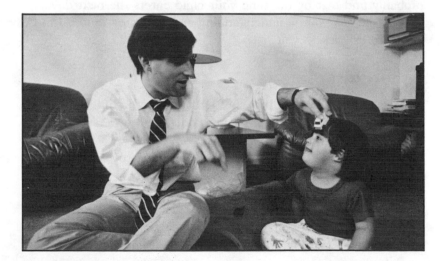

You will notice that she is interested in helping you when you dress her. She can be most cooperative. She is also very capable of taking off her shoes and socks even though she will not be able to put them back on. Encourage these self-help skills. After all, your goal is to turn your toddler into a full-fledged adult. These early signs of independence are to be encouraged.

You are still the main source of receptive language building for your child. You'll want to begin to use more specific and descriptive words for things. Talk about how things taste, how they feel, and the sounds that things make. You'll want to talk about shapes, sizes, and colors. Remember that her receptive language is more highly developed than her expressive language. You can feel comfortable using words like "fuchsia" for "pink" and "huge" for "big." Talking about foods in a positive way gives your little one the idea that all foods are acceptable and may prevent some of her "I hate spinach" attitudes. "These peas are a glowing green color." Using exciting and descriptive words doesn't mean that you want to bury your toddler in an avalanche of words. Keep your phrases short and directly related to objects and activities around your child.

At this age you will see a great increase in your child's expressive language. She is making even more rapid gains in her receptive language and you can help her with this by keeping your phrases short. Don't be afraid to repeat the same words over and over; your child learns by hearing the same words again and again. You will probably find that by the time your child enters the next developmental age she will be understanding and repeating more of those same words back to you.

Fisher-Price Garage

You and your child probably spend a lot of time in the car together, especially if you are seeing doctors, teachers, and therapists. You can add those experiences to your play with this toy. This is when children begin to understand that toys represent life in many ways. You can talk about how the doctor has a garage at his office building. Perhaps you go up the ramp at that garage and come down in the elevator. By relating her real life experiences to her play experiences, you can help her understand more about those events. Children enjoy pretend play. We will discuss a few of the

Fisher-Price representational toys such as the farm, the school, and the house but you may want to purchase others or share with a friend.

Some of the language concepts that can be taught with the garage are:

up the elevator
down the ramp
turn the handle
stop and go
fill the cars with gas
put the driver in the car

Here's how the play might go:

> ...Let's get all of our cars out. Can you find the blue car? Good, now where's the green one? Okay, show me the yellow car. Now what color is the last one? You're right, it's red. What color is our car? You're right, our car is blue. Let's put the red car into the elevator. Here it goes up, up, up. (If you pause here your toddler will probably imitate you in saying 'up.') Now the red car is at the top. Let's find the red parking space so we can park the car. Good, you found the red space and you put the red car in the right spot. Let's go back down, down, down the elevator and find the blue one. Put the blue car in the elevator. Listen to the bell as the car goes up. Ding, ding, ding. Here we are at the top. Can you find the blue parking space?...

Single Concept

Can you find the *red* car? Yes, that's *red* just like your shirt. Let's put the *red* car into the elevator. Now the *red* car is at the top. Let's find the *red* parking space so we can park our *red* car. Good, you found the *red* space. You even put the *red* car in the *red* parking spot. Great job!

Continue in this way until all of the cars are parked. Then you can ride each of the men up in the side of the elevator and put them into their cars.

...Well, now everyone is in their car. Where do you think the driver of the blue car wants to go? That's a good idea. Maybe he wants to go home for supper. Let's drive the blue car to the ramp. Here we go. Brrrrr. Oooooooo down the ramp. Off he goes. He's going home for supper now. What about the driver of the yellow car? Uh oh, she just noticed that she needs some gas. There's a gas pump at the bottom of the ramp. Shall we drive down the ramp? Let's hear you now—Ooooooo down the ramp. (Encourage this vocalization from your toddler). Get the gas pump. Put the gas into the car. Now the car has some gas in it. Where do you think the driver wants to go? Maybe she needs to go to the grocery store to get some food for dinner. Off she goes....

Continue in this way, creating new and different places for each driver to go. If your child has the language, she can contribute her ideas and her places to your play. You may have ideas of what you want to do but follow her lead when she wants to play in a certain way. You can give her whatever language she needs for the scenes that she will create. Even though we describe a lot of talking on your part, we encourage you to pause at certain times to allow her to imitate you or for her to tell you what her ideas are.

On the bottom floor of the garage is a stop sign that you can raise and lower as the cars come in and out. This is a nice time to

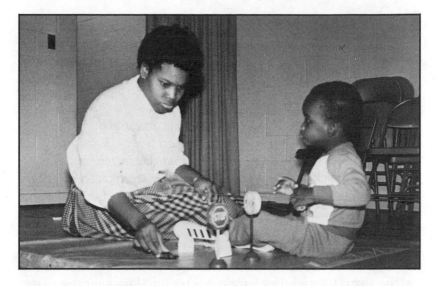

introduce the ideas of stop and go. You can be the traffic director and say "stop" and "go" when appropriate and then you can switch jobs and let your toddler be the traffic controller. When you are driving in the car, be sure to point out stop signs that look like the one in the toy and that they mean stop. You can involve your passenger by telling her to let you know when it's okay to "go." Of course, you will be sure to check for yourself. This can carry over to traffic lights as well. While you are stopped for a red light you can tell her that red means "stop" and green means "go." She can help you watch for the green light and tell you that it's okay to go now. These car activities keep your child alert and involved. They also provide excellent language input time.

Single Concept

Look, Michelle. Here's a green light. What does the green light mean? Right! It means we can *go*. See the car in front of us? It is *going* now. Now we can *go* too. A green light means *go*. Do you think that car will *go* now? Yes, it can *go* now. It has a green light. See it *go*.

Special Considerations

If your child is visually impaired, you may want to introduce the concept of listening to traffic for clues as to what is happening.

Unimax Zoo Set

We hope that you live in an area that has a zoo. Before and after your trip you can use the Unimax Zoo Set to talk about what you will see at the zoo. The animals that are in this set are the panda, cat, camel, giraffe, lion, hippo, zebra, elephant, and tiger. There are bags of plastic animals that you can find in the toy store that you can add to this set.

Additionally there is a zoo keeper, a tree, a signboard, and a jeep with a trailer. There are also six sections of fencing so you can build enclosures for the animals. Talking about each of the animals and the characteristics they have is always fun. Plan your trip to the zoo so that you can see one or two of the animals in the zoo set. Probably because of their size, elephants have always been fascinating for youngsters. Seeing a real one and feeding it peanuts is an experience most children and adults enjoy. Watching an elephant reach out with his long trunk is fascinating. You can reenact this experience with your play set at home.

> ...Let's build a fence for the elephant. Can you find the elephant? Good for you. Put the elephant inside of the fence. We have to be careful because he is *sooooo* big. Look at his long trunk. Do you remember yesterday when we saw a real elephant at the zoo? Remember how long his trunk was! This is a toy elephant—he has a long trunk too. What color is the elephant? We saw a gray elephant at the zoo yesterday. Let's take the elephant out of the fence. Who do you want to play with now?...

With each animal you can talk about his eyes, nose, mouth, tail, teeth, and other exotic things about them. You can introduce the zoo keeper and talk about the jobs that she does. You can put her on the jeep and put one of the animals in the trailer to drive it over to the zoo enclosure. Remember to talk about things you saw at the zoo and relate them to the animals in the toy zoo. Your toddler should be able to imitate and even initiate some of the words that you arc using here.

Single Concept

This elephant is a *big* animal. Did you see the *big* animal at the zoo yesterday? Do you see another *big* animal here? You're right. The giraffe is *big*. Is the panda *big?* No. What is this animal? A camel? Right. Yes, the camel is *big* too. The camel we saw at the zoo was *bigger* than this camel. Let's put all the *big* animals together. We have a lot of *big* animals here. Great, you found another *big* animal.

Mattel Zoo See 'N Say

To go along with your zoo play and zoo visit, consider the Mattel See 'N Say toy. A word about these toys in general. They are pull voice toys: that is you pull a string and a voice tells you something about the pictures on the front of the toy. To operate this toy you turn a pointer until it points to a picture, then you pull the string and the voice talks about the picture. You must be careful to turn the pointer around several times and then point to the picture because otherwise it seems to get off track and while you're busily telling your toddler what to listen for, it will talk about something entirely different.

In the Zoo See 'N Say, the following animals are represented: elephant, lion, monkey, wolf, kangaroo, seal, tiger, hyena, zebra, panda, parrot, hippo. It is a fun toy for talking about the different animals. Sometimes the zoo keeper will make the sound of the animal while for others he will talk about a characteristic.

The pull string on this toy is not very easy for a young child to operate. She will often pull the string only halfway which will give her only half of the message. We suggest you wait until she is a little older before giving it to her to play with alone. It may be too frustrating for her at this age for it to be an independent toy.

We suggest books at the end of this section that you will also want to use with your child to talk about the zoo and animals. You can use the books both before and after the zoo trip.

Special Considerations

Once again, the quality of sound on this toy will not be clear enough for a hearing impaired child. We encourage you, however, not to abandon it entirely but to use it when your child can lipread you as well as listen. If your child has a visual impairment you will want to reinforce her listening with a vivid description of the animal that the zoo keeper is talking about.

Fisher-Price Telephone Walkie Talkie

During this developmental age, language includes babbling turning into jargon with about 25 true words thrown in. This is a stage of increased interest in talking and toy telephones are wonderful for encouraging talking and babbling. For many years, we have seen toddlers "talking" on a variety of toy telephones. We were pleased to see the Fisher-Price Telephone Walkie Talkie version of the telephone which we think your child will find highly motivating. These walkie talkies are built to look like "princess" phones. You can actually have a conversation with your child that she can hear through the phones.

You can initiate any type of conversation. You can pretend to call Dad or Mom at the office and have a conversation about what you have done that day. You can use the telephone walkie talkie to practice speech exercises of babbling and sound imitation. You can use the phones as a medium for asking the child to point to certain items that you are using for language teaching. "Show me your eyes." "Point to your mouth." "Where is your nose?"

It is a fun way of stimulating your child to talk. You will also see when she is left alone with the toy that there will be a lot of jargoning and babbling going on as she imitates what she sees you doing when you talk on the phone.

Special Considerations

Of course, if your child has a profound hearing impairment, the quality of sounds of these phones may not be sufficient for her to hear through them. This doesn't mean you shouldn't use this toy but we suggest that you play with it where your child can see you as well as try to use her residual hearing.

Bubbles

Bubbles are great fun at any age. They are a wonderful speech practice tool. Toddlers love to chase the bubbles and we have found that it may be the only way to elicit "voice" from some children as they get into the carefree "pop pop" of popping the bubbles. You can buy bubbles very inexpensively at lots of stores. Once you have the container and the bubble wand, you can continue the fun by mixing your own bubbles in the same container. Fill the jar three quarters full with water. Add about 3-4 squirts of dishwashing detergent and you're back in business again.

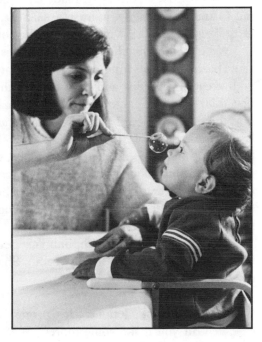

At first you may want to blow the bubbles yourself. Small children often lack the breath control to do it themselves. They will enjoy running about and popping the bubbles. Try having her imitate "pop" as she pops the bubble. As in any speech game, accept whatever sound she gives you and model the correct way for her. Give her the opportunity to try to blow the bubbles also. When she blows too hard, take her arm and blow gently on it. She will feel the difference between a gentle stream of air and a hard one. You will just love her face the first time that she is successful at getting a good stream of bubbles out. We have never seen a child who was not fascinated with this activity. You may also find that your older child will enjoy blowing bubbles with her younger brother or sister.

Be careful that your youngster does not swallow the bubbly water as she puts her mouth close to the wand to blow it. Do not leave her unattended with the jar of bubbles. You also may want to do this outside or on a floor that can be mopped. It is inevitable that the bubble mixture will spill! Even if it doesn't spill, if you play for a long time you will have a soapy film on the floor and furniture.

Soapy Sails Bath Toy

This sturdy, colorful toy, made by Colorform, has many appealing features—a bear, a walrus, a sailboat, a tugboat. Perhaps the most exciting feature is a flag that makes bubbles when it is moved.

We talked about the magic of bubbles earlier. You can use the same basic dialogues for the flag bubbler too. Children are enchanted with creating bubbles and they can do this by simply turning the flag. You can encourage your child to make the bubbles and then pop them. Introduce the concept of *all gone* and *disappeared* as the last of the stream of bubbles drifts away. Talk about how the bubbles go "up, up, up" and then back "down, down, down." Show your child how they "blow away." She might enjoy crouching down and directing the stream of bubbles with her breath. This is a great exercise for any language delayed child who needs work on getting more breath behind some of her sounds.

Kids are fascinated with bubbles because they disappear as quickly and mysteriously as they came. Share the excitement of this mystery with your child.

...Look, Jennifer. It's magic. They're all gone. Can you make some more?...

The bubbles are also great for describing shape, size, and color as well as working on counting skills.

...The bubbles are round. Can you see the circles? Look, there's a big bubble. See all the beautiful colors! They're pink, and blue, and what else? That's right! Purple. And that one's clear. It

has no color at all and you can see right through it.
Let's see how many bubbles you can make. Wow!
You made so many! One...two...three....

Homemade Toys

Tape Recorder

Our suggestion for a homemade toy for this age group is not exactly a toy. We suggest a tape recorder and some tapes. Fisher-Price has a children's tape recorder which has very good sound reproduction and is very sturdy. There are also excellent tapes available in stores. You can buy them or make them. We suggest some tapes that you will want to make with and for your child.

First, we highly recommend that you tape your child's expressive language periodically throughout her life. Start with those very early coos and babbles. Can you imagine her surprise when you play them for her when she is older? Second, we suggest that you tape her on each of her birthdays. Once again this is a wonderful remembrance to treasure.

In addition to taping her expressive language, tape stories that she likes to listen to. In this way, she can turn on her tape recorder and listen to you tell a story while she turns the pages. On our recordings we tape a reading of the story with our children participating. For example, we might be reading a Dr. Seuss book. When it comes to a part that is repeated, we stop reading and have our child say the refrain part. We also pause when it is time to turn the page and have our child say, "Turn the page." When she is alone with this tape, she can "read" the book with the tape and turn the page when she is told to do so.

At this early age, use very short and very simple books. Some examples are books that have one object on the page. Your child can "read" the object and then say "Turn the page." She can then listen to herself later with the book.

If you enjoy music, you may want to sing a few songs alone or with your child and tape them for her to listen to later on.

If your child has a hearing impairment, do not abandon this idea entirely but use it for auditory training lessons when encouraging her to listen for specific things. You might want to have three toys in front of her and have the tape ask her for a specific one. That way she will be depending only on her residual hearing and may surprise you with what she is able to pick up this way. It is also good practice for taking hearing tests where she is expected to respond to sound that she does not see. You might say on this tape, "Put the block in the box," or "Put the ring on the cone," and this will help train her for hearing tests.

Styrofoam Boats

Save the styrofoam plates that meat and fish come on in the supermarket. You can cut a triangle from a piece of paper, stick a toothpick through it and stick it into the styrofoam to make a boat. You can use this for practicing blowing skills which can help teach your child breath control. You can float the boats in a tub, sink, or outdoor small pool. You and your child can have a race with each other, each of you blowing your boat to the finish line. Sometimes it helps a young child to direct her breath if you have her use a straw to blow through. That will concentrate whatever breath she has in a straight line. Some children find this fun and get better results than just blowing wildly about.

Eighteen To Twenty-Four Months

As your toddler nears the developmental age of two years, you will notice an incredible leap in his expressive language. If you remember our discussion on language development, we talked about how he will probably have almost three hundred words by the end

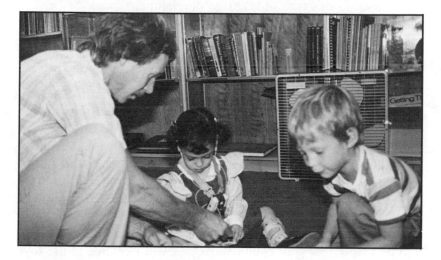

of this time frame. All of the hard work that you have put in will be worth it as you hear him come out with more and more recognizable words.

This is where your months of playing imitation games will begin to make sense. You don't want to correct your child when he says phrases incorrectly or uses the wrong tenses of verbs. What you want to do is model the correct way to say them and hope that he will want to imitate you. When he says, "car go me," you say, "OK, you want to go in the car, we're leaving soon."

Remember that you are continuing to build your child's receptive language at the same time that you're admiring his growing expressive language. Reading books, playing with him and with his toys, and using descriptive and novel words are great activities for this age. While you are looking at books together, involve him in the "telling of the story" by asking him questions about the pictures he sees.

His love of jumping at this age may spell big trouble for your bed and his. Do you have an old mattress? Put it in his playroom and let him jump about to his heart's content. Put his indoor slide next to it so he can slide down onto a soft place. Having an indoor slide gives you a lot of opportunity for language input of action words and prepositions like "up," "down," and "under." He is ready to learn this now and you can count on his love of active play to stimulate his interest in this type of language development.

Outside he needs a fenced area or you need to be with him. This is the time when you can begin talking about cars and setting limits of where he can play. Don't expect him to follow these rules without supervision. He is endlessly curious and may set off in any direction at any time. If you have a driveway, tell him that he can go to the end of the driveway and stop. You may want to put some type of barrier up there to visually remind him. You can line your trash cans up across the drive. If you have a sidewalk in front of your house, he can play on *your* sidewalk but not the neighbors'. Once again, a trash can at either end of the boundary will help to remind him. If he moves beyond those boundaries, you will be there to gently remind him of the rule.

The toys we suggest in this section, as in every other section, can be adapted for your child's language level. Feel free to use toys from other sections if they seem more appropriate to you.

Take advantage of his energy level and take a trip to the park. There you'll find many physical activity toys such as slides, swings, and seesaws which provide great opportunity for language building. We urge you *just* to use the language that you think of as you push your child up and down on the swings and as he goes way up in the air on the seesaw or round and round on the merry-go-round.

> ...You want to go on the swing now? Okay, up you go. Let's put this bar down so you don't slip out. Here we go. (If this is a new experience for your child, stay in front of the swing and gently push it back and forth.) You're swinging now. The swing goes back and forth, back and forth. You're swinging. Back you go and forward you come. Back and

forth. You're swinging! Do you want to go higher? Up you go. Down you come. Up and down.

This is the seesaw. When you go up, Johnny goes down. (If this is the first time for your child to go on the seesaw, stay on his side with him. If you have no playmate for the other end, you can make it go up and down by pushing him down and lifting his side up.) Here you go, up in the air. Look how high you are. You are up in the air. Shall we go down? Down, down, down. Now you are back on the ground again. You came down. Do you want to go up again? Up, up, up; way up high. And now it's down, down, down again.

Let's try the merry-go-round. It goes round and round. (If you're not sure that your child will stay seated, sit with him on your lap and push the merry-go-round with your feet.) Round and round and round we go. Everything is spinning by. We're going round and round and round. Close your eyes. Can you still feel us going round and round? Oooh, I feel a little dizzy. Sometimes you feel dizzy going round and round...

Indoor Slides

Many different companies make indoor slides. One word of caution: make sure that the spaces between the steps are either wide enough or small enough that a small head cannot get stuck between them. Make sure that it is sturdily built and that there are no pieces that could splinter.

One favorite teaching activity with this toy is to have a child wait at the bottom of the ladder for you to say "up" as he climbs each step. This is an excellent exercise for teaching waiting his turn and if he is hearing impaired, it is an easy auditory training game. The word "up" has a lot of auditory energy and is easy for even a profoundly hearing impaired child to hear. When you have done "up" for the steps, have him wait at the top for the command "down." It is fun to expand this game to a stuffed toy or doll. Your child can then give the command to his stuffed friend which will help him with his expressive language as well as allowing him to control the game. When you get to the "down" part of the activity, you can add in a long vowel sound for the sliding part—"oooooo down."

In the indoor slide there is also a space under the slide where you can talk about the concept of *under*. The prepositions "in," "on," "under," "behind," and "in front of" can all be taught using this slide. You can give directions to your child to go under the slide, stand behind it, or in front of it. If your child is afraid to do these ac-

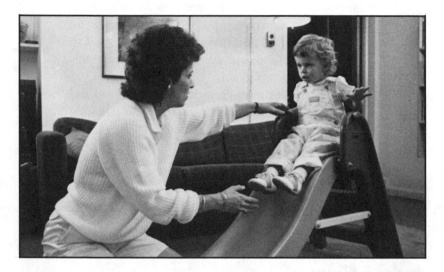

tivities, you can have stuffed animals go on the slide or in the hole. You can also kneel in front of the slide and extend your arms to him as he comes down the slide.

> ...Do you want to go up the slide? Stand here at the bottom and listen. When I say 'up,' you go up one step. Okay, up you go. Good—wait. Okay, up again. One more. Up you go. Now you're at the top. Sit down and get ready to slide down. Listen. Okay, down you go. Wheeee, down you go...

It is fun to take small cars and have them ride down the slide also. Matchbox makes many small replicas of different kinds of cars and you can use the appropriate names for each of the cars.

...Look, I have some cars here. Let's put them at the top of the slide. Here's a van and a Chevy. Which do you want? Okay, I'll take the Chevy. Let's make them go down the slide. Are you ready? Go! They went down the slide. Down to the bottom. Shall we do it again? Go and get the cars...

An extra benefit is that the slide is an active toy for a toddler and will help him use up some of his excess energy in very positive ways.

Puzzles

Puzzles range from very simple to incredibly complex. The primary skills that they teach are eye/hand coordination and the ability to visualize abstract shapes. At their very simplest, they consist of one object-one space types of puzzles. There are fine ones made out of wood that have knobs to aid in lifting the pieces out of the puzzle as well as placing them back in. We recommend the wooden ones since they are very sturdy and your child can use the pieces in a variety of other play situations without fear of damaging the pieces.

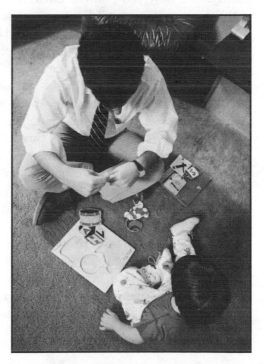

Puzzles increase in complexity until you reach adulthood where there are hundreds and thousands of small pieces and very complicated designs. When our children were small, we always had a puzzle out on a table where anyone passing by could add a piece or two. We often sat together at the table and TV was quickly forgotten when we were spurred on by someone finding just the right piece of blue sky. It is a great family activity for people of all ages.

The puzzles we recommend for this age group are the very simplest, with one piece-one space concepts. You can find these in any toy store. The one we describe is made by Playskool and has the following pieces in it: a clown doll, a pull toy duck, a teddy bear, and a jack-in-the box. The clown doll is ideal for reviewing those good ol' body parts. Now you will see the receptive language that you have been building come out in expressive language.

> ...Show me the doll's eyes. Can you say 'eyes'?
> Where are the doll's ears? Can you show me your
> ears? Let me hear you say 'ear.'...

And so on for the rest of the facial parts.

After you have finished talking about the clown doll, put that puzzle piece out of sight. Next take out the pull toy duck. You can demonstrate how you pull the duck. You can talk about the color of the duck and check to see if your child knows the color yellow. The actual speech production of this word is often difficult for young children so don't rush to jump in to correct his speech. Remember our modeling behavior. Just repeat back, "You're right—that's a *yellow* duck" with a slight pause and slight emphasis on the word, *yellow*. You can talk about how the duck swims in water and says "quack, quack." These are fun babbling types of sounds for your youngster to imitate. Be sure to mention that the duck has feathers and ask your youngster if *he* has feathers. As with the doll, put the duck away after you have finished talking about it.

Next take out the teddy bear. Of course, your child has his own teddy bear and you might have it on hand so that you can compare the toys. The puzzle teddy bear is hard and the toy teddy bear is soft. Then you can go back to some of those textures that we talked about many months ago. The puzzle teddy is smooth and the toy teddy is furry. Use as many expressive words as you can think of. Once again you have the opportunity to talk about facial and body parts. This young person is really going to be ready for all of those standardized tests that ask for recognition of body parts! You might want to practice on some action verbs by having the teddy bear *jump, run, walk, hide,* and *sleep.* When you have finished talking about the bear, put it out of sight with the other two pieces.

You are now ready for the final piece, which is the jack-in-the-box.

...This puzzle piece is smaller than this jack-in-the-box. Where's Jack? When Jack comes out of the box, he *pops* up. Hi, Jack! See Jack's hat? Jack has a big nose. Do you see Jack's nose? Where is your nose? Right! Where is Mommy's nose?...

Once again, put Jack with all of the other puzzle pieces. Now is the time to "test" your child's receptive language of these pieces. Put out two at a time and ask him to choose which one you are talking about. At first you might just ask for the toy.

...Which is the clown doll? Where is the yellow duck? Give me the piece that pops up. Which is the teddy bear?...

After you have played with this puzzle a few times, you might put two pieces in front of your child and ask him a riddle.

...This piece has soft and fuzzy fur and you like to sleep with him at night...

Then have him choose between the two pieces. Build this up until you can lay all four of the puzzle pieces out and have him choose the one that you are describing. If he has the expressive ability to tell you about the pieces, even if it is just the name, have *him* be the "teacher" and ask you to find the one that he is talking about. Remember that he will probably have quite a bit of expressive language at this point and this is a fun way for him to use it. If his speech production is poor, you can model it correctly when you "find" the piece that he is asking for. You can say, "I found that *teddy bear,*" pausing ever so slightly to emphasize the correct way to say the word.

When you really get going on these puzzles, you can do two at the same time and have him choose from among eight puzzles. We know one toddler who used to dump all twelve of her puzzles in a heap on the floor and scoot about from puzzle to puzzle fitting in the pieces.

As we said in the beginning, puzzles are a great way to teach a lot of vocabulary. There are beginning single piece-single space puzzles that have as many as thirty small objects to be placed. We suggest that if you use these that you start by only removing one row at a time to avoid confusion with too many pieces.

Fisher-Price Farm

The Fisher-Price Farm has twenty-two pieces. There are four people, including the farmer, as well as a dog, cow, sheep, pig, horse, rooster, hen, silo, fence, barn, and tractor. The vocabulary for the animals would consist of their physical characteristics as well as their sounds and what they eat.

Dog–eyes, nose, mouth, tail, ears, four paws, arf-arf, bark, helps the farmer round up the sheep and cows, eats dog food or table scraps.

>...Can you find the dog? Does he look like your dog? Well, some things are the same and some are

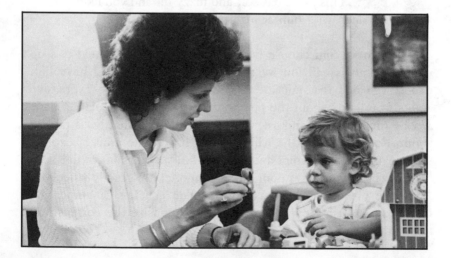

different. He has a tail–can you find his tail? Good.
That's right. That's his tail. (Continue with each of
the body parts.) Do you know what the dog eats?
On the farm he probably eats all the leftover food
from the table. What does our dog eat? You're
right–he eats dog food from a can...

Cow– eyes, nose, mouth, tail, ears, udders, hooves, moos, eats
grass, the farmer gets milk from the cow to make cheese and
butter.

> ...Where's the cow? Did you see the cow yester-
> day when we went to the farm? This is a toy cow
> but she has the same parts as the cow on the farm.
> Look for the tail. Can you find it? (Go through all
> the body parts, labeling them if necessary.) The
> farmer gets milk from the cow. Some of the milk
> he gives to his family and other milk comes to us
> in the grocery store. The milk we drink comes from
> the cow...

Sheep–eyes, nose, mouth, short stubby tail, wooly coat, hooves,
baa, eats grass, gives us wool to make sweaters and other clothing.

> ...Here's the sheep. The sheep is very fluffy.
> You know the farmer cuts the sheep's wool when it
> gets very long and makes yarn from it. Do you know
> what we do with the yarn? We make sweaters with
> the yarn. The sweaters are warm because wool is
> warm. When the sheep gets his wool cut, new wool
> will grow back. One sheep can make lots of warm
> sweaters for us...

Go through the sheep's body parts and compare them with the
body parts of the other animals.

Horse—eyes, nose, mouth, long swishing tail, ears, hooves, can pull the plow, helps the farmer with planting, the farmer can ride on the horse, the horse gallops, trots, runs, neighs, eats hay, or grains.

> ...A farmer always needs a horse on the farm. The horse is very strong and can help him pull heavy loads. The farmer can put all the hay in the wagon and then the horse can pull the heavy wagon all the way back to the barn. Do you remember when you rode on a horse at the park?...

Rooster—is the daddy of the chickens, wakes up the farmer early in the morning, cock-a-doodle-do, has a red "comb" on the top of his head, eyes, beak, eats corn.

> ...Here's a rooster. He wakes everyone up in the morning. Listen to the sound he makes. 'Cock-a-doodle-do.' Now it's your turn. Can you wake up the farmer in the morning with 'cock-a-doodle-do?' You woke him up...

Hen—is the mommy of the chickens, feathers, eyes, beak, eats corn, cluck, cluck, gives eggs to the farmer.

> ...This is a little hen. Do you know that the hen is the animal that gives us the eggs that we have for breakfast? The hen lays eggs. The farmer collects the eggs. Some he keeps for his family and he sells the rest to the grocery stores so that we can buy them for our breakfast. What kind of eggs do you like to eat? You like scrambled eggs. Daddy likes soft-boiled eggs, and I like hard-boiled eggs. The eggs come from the hen on the farm...

You can talk about all the different farm buildings as you set up the farm.

Barn–All of the animals sleep in the barn, there is hay in the barn, there is a loft in the barn. When you open the barn door on this toy, it makes kind of a creaking sound–many barn doors creak.

> ...The barn is a very important building for all the animals on the farm. The barn is where all of the animals sleep at night. The cow sleeps in the barn. The horse sleeps in the barn. Do you know what other animals sleep in the barn? That's right, the dog and the sheep sleep in the barn too. The barn helps them stay warm and dry....

Tractor–The farmer drives the tractor to make rows for the crops that he plants. Talk about the big wheels of the tractor and the sounds it makes as it drives around.

> ...This is the tractor that the farmer drives. He uses it to make rows when he is getting ready to plant. What do you think he will plant this year? Maybe he will plant rows of corn. Do you like to eat corn? The farmer uses the tractor to help him make the rows nice and straight. The tractor has very big wheels because it goes into the fields and the wheels keep it from getting stuck in the mud. Did you see the big wheels on the tractor at the farm?...

Silo–This is where all of the extra grain is kept. Talk about harvest time and keeping some of the grain for the winter when there is no crop. Talk about seasons and how they are different.

> ...Do you know what this tall building is called? It's called a silo. The farmer keeps all the extra grain in this building during the winter. In the spring, the farmer plants all the seeds. The seeds make different foods in the summer. After all the food grows, the farmer will collect all that food. Some of the

food he will keep for himself and his family. Some he will sell to supermarkets, and the rest he will keep in this silo. That way, during the winter he will have food for his animals. In the winter nothing grows so he has to save food. What should we save in our silo? Shall we keep extra wheat and extra corn? Since we planted corn with our tractor, maybe we'll keep the extra corn in our silo....

Fence–The rooster and hen are made so that they can sit on the fence. You can put animals behind the fence, in front of the fence, or in the fenced in section.

> ...Do you remember seeing the big fence around the farm yesterday? Why do you think the farmers need to have a fence. The farmer needs a fence to keep all his animals inside the farm. The cows and sheep might wander away if there were no fence. Let's build a fence around our barn and silo. Now, let's put all the animals inside the fence. Can you find the sheep? Put it inside the fence. Now, where's the cow? Put it inside the fence. The horse needs to go inside the fence also. Where are the hen and the rooster? Let's put them inside the fence. Good! Now all the animals are inside the fence....

Of course, we suggest that you and your youngster go out to visit a farm. Many areas of the country have working farms that will welcome your visit. If you call ahead most farmers will be willing to spend a few minutes with you and let your youngster touch the animals and watch them being fed or milked. As we know, the more hands-on experiences that he has, the better. Nothing reinforces learning like actually doing the things you are learning about.

Unimax also makes a farm set and if you have both you can add them together at play time. This would make it more realistic because farms rarely have only one of each animal as these sets do.

You might also be able to purchase small farm animals in bags with many animals in each.

In our book section, we suggest several books that talk about farm animals to reinforce what you have seen, touched, and played with.

Mattel See 'N Say—The Farmer Says

This toy is almost exactly the same as the Zoo See 'N Say described before. This time farm animals are represented and the farmer talks about the sounds that the animals make. The animals that the farmer talks about are:

cat	horse
turkey	coyote
sheep	pig
dog	rooster
duck	cow
frog	bird

The sounds that come from this toy are remarkably good. The same caution applies to pulling the string. Make sure you have turned the pointer several times and then pull the string all in one motion. You may find that your youngster is more capable of doing this at this age then he was earlier but he still may need your help.

Special Considerations

If your child has a hearing impairment the quality of the sound will probably not be sufficient for him to hear it. Don't ignore the toy. Tell him beforehand what he will hear and then have him listen for it. He should be able to tell you the name of the animals because he will see which one the pointer is pointing to so that he can always "guess" correctly.

Washing And Grooming Activity

Toddlers love to help you wash and dress them. They are showing the first signs of wanting to do things for themselves. You can take advantage of this desire, add it to his lengthened attention span, and come up with the Scrub 'N Fun Center by Fisher-Price. You could easily use Walt Disney's Mickey Mouse Wash and Play

Grooming Center by Illco Toys instead. Since this is the time when your child will probably go to get his first haircut, you can fit that experience into your dialogues with whatever toy you choose to use.

> ...Time to go to the beauty parlor, just like Mommy. First, we wash your hair. Let's get some shampoo. Now we'll pour the shampoo on your hair. Look in the mirror. See the soap bubbles? We're getting your hair all clean....

Most kids are not terribly thrilled about having their hair washed because the soap and water drips into their eyes. Try to get your toddler to "help" wash his own hair. This will help him feel as if he is doing something for himself. Once he has tired of "washing," you go on to do the job as quickly as possible. You can distract him with some of the other features of this toy.

> ...Where are the cups? Oh, I see them. One is green, and there is the yellow one. Can you fill them up? Push down on the faucet. Use two hands. Here, I'll help you. Now set them on this ledge....

Have your child rinse his hair with the toy shower head. He may enjoy the light stream of water trickling down his body as long as he feels he has some control over the amount of water. Give your child some appropriate language to describe the sensation he is feeling.

> ...You're spraying yourself with water. Doesn't that feel nice? I bet that tickles a little. Can you spray Mom's hand? Now I'm wet too. Now let's spray your arm...foot...knee....

Before you wind up bath time for the day, give him a chance to enjoy combing and brushing his hair with the miniature grooming set.

> ...Here's the brush. You can brush your hair.
> Here. Mommy will help. Now let's put the brush
> back in its holder. Say goodbye to the little boy
> (point to your child's reflection in the mirror on the
> toy). Time to leave the beauty parlor. We'll come
> back tomorrow....

Your child will not outgrow this toy in a hurry. For the next few years he will enjoy experimenting with it in new and different ways. We suggest you keep it in the tub until he begins to lose interest. But by all means don't put it away forever. His interest will re-emerge every few months as he becomes increasingly independent and more eager to do things for himself.

Homemade Toys

Mini Sandbox

The homemade toy we recommend is a sandbox made from a plastic shoe box. We feel plastic is best because it will hold up longer than a cardboard box. You can vary what you use for "sand." You can use sand, dried beans, or rice. The material doesn't really matter and if you want to, you can even have one of each. The idea here is to provide a toy that your child can use to:

fill	spill
pour	turn over
empty	squeeze
dump	pile
measure	top
touch	

Your play with this toy may go something like this:

> ...Oh, it's raining out today. Let's play with your
> indoor sandbox. Let's go find it. Here's a cup. Can
> you fill it all the way to the top? Good job, Jeff—the
> cup is full. You want to pour it out? Okay, pour it
> out—ooooooooooo all gone now. Now your cup is

> empty. Look, Jeff here's a funnel. Let's fill up this
> milk bottle with sand. Can you fill it half full with
> sand? Whoops—stop there. It's half full now. You
> dumped it out. Now the bottle is empty. What shall
> we fill up now?...

Your role is to provide the language for the activity that he is involved with by cueing words or repeating.

Pretend Painter's Set

Another homemade toy for this age group which your child will love is designed to be used in the bathtub or wading pool. Quite simply, you can create a pretend painter's set for your child by providing him with a wide paintbrush (at least 2 inches wide) and a plastic pail filled with water. Your child's fine motor skills have developed to the point where he can easily hold onto and paint with a brush of this size, and he will take great pride in painting "all by himself."

Encourage your child's play by demonstrating how he can fill the bucket with the water from the tub, and sit the bucket upright on the inside corner of the tub so it won't spill over onto the bathroom floor. Help your child transform the water in his pail into imaginary paint by asking:

> ...What will you paint today? Does your house
> need painting? (Motion to the tiles on the inside of
> the tub.) What color will you paint your house? Dip
> your brush into the bucket. Get your brush all wet.
> There now, you're ready to begin. I wonder what
> you will paint today?...

With this Pretend Painter's Set, you can let your child paint to his heart's content, and not have to worry about the water causing any permanent damage. We have found this game can occupy a child's interest because it is so relaxing and so much fun.

Vocabulary And Concepts

The following list will give you an idea of the vocabulary and concepts that your child should be familiar with.

action words (dump, measure, spill, squeeze)
behind
birthday
bubbles
Disney characters (Mickey Mouse, Dumbo, Goofy, Pluto,
    Donald Duck)
farm animals (rooster, hen)
farm equipment (barn, tractor)
give me the
in front of
names of cars
nursery rhymes
opposites (before/after, push/pull, short/tall, big/little)
playground equipment (swing, slide, seesaw, merry-go-round)
prepositions (under, over, in, on)
put it in
self help skills (getting dressed, going to the potty, brush
    hair, wash hair, eating meals)
shapes (round, circle, square, triangle)
sharing
show me the
take it out
taking turns
transportation (boat, car, airplane, train)
weather
what
when
where
who
where is the
zoo animals (bear, hippo, rhino)

Toy Summary

The following is a list of the toys we used for this developmental age. The * indicates a homemade toy.

bubbles	Soapy Sails Bath Toy
Fisher-Price Farm	Surprise box
Fisher-Price Garage	Unimax Zoo Set
Fisher-Price	Washing and Grooming Water
Walkie Talkie	Toy
Floating Family	*large boxes
water toy	*Playdough
indoor slide	*pretend painter's set
Mattel Zoo See 'N Say	*sandboxes and sand toys
Mattel See 'N Say–	*styrofoam boats
The Farmer Says	*tape recorder and tapes
push toys	
pull toys	
puzzles	

Books

Your child will enjoy books if you spend time reading with him every day. Books that name things are still his favorites. Now he should be able to name more and more of the pictures in his old favorites. Books should be added to and never put away so that they can be enjoyed again and again. He also will be able to follow a simple story plot at this time. Some of the picture books that have no words are also fun.

Since we have visited the zoo, we suggest several zoo animal books. You can read these both before you go and after you have been to the zoo. Other titles you might be interested in also focus on animals. Be sure to choose others that you see in the library when you visit.

Remember your language books that you made a while back? You can take pictures on your farm or zoo visit and add this to your language experience books. If you have a Polaroid camera, you can have instant pictures and you can make the book the same day. At this age when you make a language book, have your child give you the language for each picture. Then you write what he says. It's wonderful to look back at these books as your children get older.

Animals in the Zoo, Feodor Rojankavosky, New York: Knopf, 1962.
A beautiful alphabet book that features different zoo animals for each letter. A good book to read both before and after a visit to the zoo.

Ask Mr. Bear, Marjorie Flack, New York: Macmillan, 1932.
An older book that has withstood the test of time. Its repetitive simplicity has appealed to children through the years. A young boy wonders what to give his mother for her birthday. He asks many animals for their suggestions until he finds the perfect solution.

Farm Animals, Nancy Sears, New York: Random House, 1977.
Large clear pictures of familiar animals.

Gobble, Growl, Grunt, Peter Spier, New York: Zephyr, 1971.
Delightful pictures of familiar and exotic animals and the very strange sounds that they make. Great fun for you and your child to read and imitate together. Good practice for the elements of speech that are just vowel-like sounds.

Good Morning, Farm, Betty Ben Wright, illustrated by Fred Weinman, Wisconsin: Whitman Publishing Co., 1964.
Beautiful photographs showing the farm dog going around to wake everyone up and say good morning. Told in delightful rhyme.

Guess What? Roger Bester, New York: Crown Publishers, 1980.
Actual photographs of common animals. The text lists three characteristics of each animal and gives your child a chance to guess which animal they may be talking about. Animals included are horse, squirrel, duck, cow, chicken, and pig. A nice follow-up story after a farm visit.

Hi Cat, Ezra Jack Keats, New York: Young Readers Press, Inc., 1970.
Archie's new friend is a crazy cat who causes all kinds of trouble, but Willie the dog teaches him a lesson. Another fine book in the offerings from this author.

It Does Not Say Meow and Other Riddle Rhymes, Beatrice Schenk de
   Regniers, illustrated by Paul Galdone, New York: Seabury,
   1972.
   Rhyming riddles are a fun way for children to learn about the
animals and their sounds in a fun way. Learning the negative in a
positive way.

Little Blue and Little Yellow, Leo Lionni, New York: Obolensky,
   1959.
   Talks about the activities of two friends, blue and yellow, and
what happens when they are together (they make green). A fun
book to read after you do your playdough activity with your child.

Little Red Hen, Paul Galdone, New York: Seabury, 1973.
   A hardworking hen tries to get her lazy friends to help her bake
some bread. Young children get the message easily from this charming story of how they must help if they want to benefit.

Millions of Cats, Wanda Gag, New York: Coward, McCann, 1928.
   A charming book that has endured for over fifty years. An elder-
ly couple would like just one little cat to keep them company, but
making the decision is hard and lots of fun.

My Day on the Farm, Chiyoko Nakatani, New York: Crowell, 1976.
   A very simple text describing the sights, sounds, smells, and
feelings of being on a farm. A nice follow-up to a real visit.

The Napping House, Audrey Wood, illustrated by Don Wood, New
   York: Harcourt, 1984.
   A clever and beautiful book for young children. A cumulative
rhyme that adds a variety of sleeping people to the bed until the
surprise ending at dawn. The lighting on the page cleverly shows
the passage of time as the night turns into morning.

Play With Me, Marie Hall Ets, New York: Viking Press, 1955.
   A little girl makes friends with different animals: a frog, turtle,
chipmunk. She learns she needs to sit quietly and wait for them to
come to her. The illustrations are simply lovely and endearing.

Sam Who Never Forgets, Eve Rice, New York: Puffin Books, 1980.
   Sam is a zoo keeper who never forgets to feed all of the animals
promptly at three o'clock until one day....

Sleepy Book, Charlotte Zolotow, illustrated by Vladimir Bobri, New York: Lothrop, Lee and Shepherd, 1958.

In very few words, the text tells about how and where different animals, including boys and girls, go to sleep. A lovely bedtime favorite.

Snake In, Snake Out, Linda Banchek, illustrated by Elaine Arnold, New York: Thomas Crowell, 1978.

An unlikely trio of an old woman, a parrot, and a snake demonstrate different prepositions such as: in, out, on, up, over, off, down, under.

Talkabout Bedtime, Margaret Keen, illustrated by Harry Wingfield, England: Ladybird Books, 1977.

A lovely book that talks about every aspect of bedtime. Different kinds of beds, different people sleeping–adults as well as children. Talks about some of the noises you might hear at bedtime and jobs that people have who work at night. As in the other "Talkabout" books, there are activities for matching and finding similarities and differences.

The Three Little Pigs can be found in many collections of nursery tales. One such collection is *My First Book of Nursery Tales,* M. Mayer, illustrated by W. Joyce, New York: Random House, 1983.

A classic tale which young children enjoy. They can join in on the repetitive part of the wolf when he says, "I will huff and puff and blow your house down." Many of the modern versions have a more humane ending for the wolf than having him boil in the stew pot. Take your choice of many versions of this classic favorite.

The Very Busy Spider, Eric Carle, New York: Philomel, 1986.

Different barnyard animals try to distract an industrious spider from building his web. Children can chime in with the different animal sounds that are described here.

Wake Up and Goodnight, Charlotte Zolotow, illustrated by Leonard Weisgard, New York: Harper and Row, 1971.

A very lyrical and charming story which begins in the morning and continues through the day into the night. A book of daily activities which your child can identify with.

What Do Toddlers Do? Photographs by Debby Slier, New York: Random House, 1985.

Beautiful, clear photographs show the everyday activities of young children picking flowers, swinging, climbing, and banging on kitchen pots.

Where's My Baby, H.A. Rey, New York: Houghton Mifflin, 1943.

This little book has a foldover page on each page. Shows the mother animals and then asks the question, "Where's my baby?" The foldover flap shows the baby animal that belongs to the mother. Gives an opportunity to talk about the actual names for the babies such as calf, colt, and lamb.

The next few pages are checklists to help you evaluate how your child is progressing.

SUMMARY OF YOUR CHILD'S SECOND YEAR 12-24 MONTHS

LANGUAGE

Developmental Milestones	Date Achieved	NOT YET	PROGRESSING
uses jargon			
names objects which ones?			
uses nouns with adjectives which adjectives?			
uses subject-predicate phrases			
uses two word sentences			
can say own name			
knows at least one family member by name			
asks for food at the table			
follows one direction at a time			
hums to music			
imitates your words			
listens to rhymes			
uses pronouns which ones?			
knows about 200 words			

PHYSICAL

Developmental Milestones	Date Achieved	NOT YET	PROGRESSING
can walk alone			
can turn pages of book			
can climb stairs on all fours			
can walk sideways			
can pull a toy			
can climb onto furniture			
can feed self			
can undress self			
can scribble			
holds crayon in fist			
can run stiffly			
can build a tower of blocks how many?			
can walk up stairs holding hand or rail			
can walk down stairs holding hand or rail			
can kick a ball			
can throw large ball			
can do single piece puzzles how many pieces?			

COGNITIVE

Developmental Milestones	Date Achieved	NOT YET	PROGRESSING
can point to facial parts eyes nose mouth			
follows simple directions Give the ball to me Sit on the chair			
can name several nouns that are familiar objects table bed toy car apple			
can point to pictures show- ing different action verbs			
can match colors red green yellow blue			
develops imaginative play			
has longer attention span			
can demonstrate under- standing of prepositions in out up down			
understands math concept of "one more"			

Twenty-Four To Thirty-Six Months

The developmental period from two to three is the one in which your toddler strives to become more independent. This period is often called the "terrible twos." A few suggestions might help you ease through this time with a little less trauma for both you and your preschooler. One simple tip is not to ask a "yes" or "no" question. If you do, you are more likely to get a "no" than a "yes." A better approach is to offer two alternatives, both of which are acceptable to you which gives your youngster a feeling of control over her life. Let's look at an example of how this might work. "Would you like to have apple juice or orange juice for a snack today?" as opposed to "Do you want apple juice?" If your child responds to the first by saying, "I want a cookie," you can calmly say, "Cookies are not a choice today. Do you want apple juice or orange juice?" If you are consistent in this approach, you should experience fewer problems.

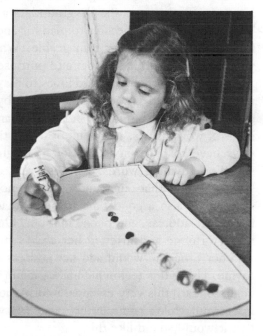

Consistency is another key issue in handling this young person. Try to establish a daily routine for her. This does not mean that it is etched in granite never to change, but as much as possible give her a routine that she can latch onto. While toddlers are struggling to become children, they also need the stability of knowing what is happening so that they feel they are in control.

Control is one of the key issues that results in misbehavior from children. Often children want to show that they are in control and parents often give up in frustration or tiredness and the children "win" again.

Keep your youngster active. She will be more likely to be demanding of your attention, fussy, and misbehave if she is bored. This doesn't mean that you need a three ring circus going all the time but try to arrange some time during each day when you have a trip to the store, the playground, or a special trip to a museum. This will give her something to plan for and give you some leverage for keeping her behavior manageable. When you do go out, keep your trip short and have a definite purpose in mind.

The two- to three-year-old loves to play rhyming games and she will learn how to use different sounds by playing these rhyming games with you. Running errands in the car is an ideal time for these kinds of word games. Just think of words that rhyme—they don't always have to make sense. A lot of laughter can come from silly sounding rhyming words. This is great exercise for all of those speech sounds that our mouth muscles need to learn to say.

This is also a good time to begin teaching your child her full name, her address, and phone number. One mother used a familiar nursery rhyme and inserted her child's full name into the rhyme. Another time she would add her address or phone number to the rhyme. Using this technique makes it fun and easy for the child to begin to learn this very essential information. For example, you can insert your child's name in the song "Mary Had A Little Lamb" so that it would sound like this:

> ...Jenny lives on Jessup Road, Jessup Road, Jessup Road, Jenny lives on Jessup Road at 12604. Jenny lives in Mt. Sinclair, Mt. Sinclair, Mt. Sinclair, Jenny lives in Mt. Sinclair, it's in the state of Maine....

Your child will love having her own personal rhyme.

You need to continue the same modeling that you have done before. Use the same idea that she has said to you but say it back to her correctly. She says, "wheel falled off"–you say, "Oh my, the wheel fell off your car. Do you need help fixing it?"

At this age, your youngster needs even more time to play alone. Many of the toys we select for this age group, are perfect for stimulating your child to create on her own.

Duplo Or Lego Blocks

These toys are ageless. We know of youngsters almost into their teens who still enjoy building intricate models with these interlocking blocks.

The beginner blocks are large, easily handled, and fit together well into tall buildings, long roads, or other fantasies created by your child. There is a time when you need to leave your child alone with these blocks as she builds creation after creation. You may sit with her later and ask her about her creation so that she has a chance to

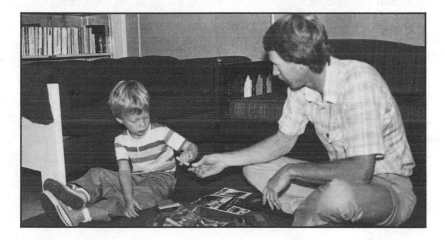

explain her fantasies. Be careful not to interject your own opinions. Do not say, "Oh, what a beautiful house you built," when, if you wait just a minute, she will tell you that she built a hotel and create stories of all of the people who are staying at the hotel. When you want to use these blocks for "teaching" language, the following ideas will be useful.

The most obvious skill to be taught is color matching and color naming. Take one block of each color–start with only two–and put them in front of you. Point to the bucket of blocks and ask her to find another blue one. When you first ask her, don't look at the blocks in front of you or indicate in any way which is blue. You are "testing" to see if she knows. If she picks up a red one or just looks at you and doesn't know which to choose, point to the blue block and say, "Can you find another one that looks just like this one?" If you still are not seeing a positive response, then pick up the blue block, rummage through the bucket, and make a big deal about finding the one that looks just like it.

> ...This is the blue one. Now we have two blue
> blocks. Look, they are the same. See this one is
> blue and this one is blue. We have two blue
> blocks....

Snap the two blocks together and go on to find another red one to match the one in front of you. When she is always successful at choosing the right color out of the bucket, you can add more blocks to the game. You should be able to quickly get to where you have all of the different colored blocks in front of you and she is able to make tall towers from them.

At another time, you will want to have your child actually name the colors as you build with them. Ask her directly, "What color is this block?" and continue until she can successfully name all of the colors that you have in your set of blocks. She may have difficulty with the naming part until a little later but asking her for the information lets her know that you expect her to learn this. Children with no delaying conditions can match and point to the correct colors by this age but often cannot "name" them themselves until a little later on.

The Duplo blocks also come with wagon type pieces that have wheels on them. You can make moving vehicles which gives you the opportunity to talk about *stop, go, wait, fast,* and *slow.* You can talk about how many wheels are on the wagon pieces and when your little builder has completed a structure, she can use it as a pull toy. If it doesn't have a string attached to the wheeled portion, it is easy enough to get a long shoelace and make your own pull string.

Other concepts you can teach with her toy are:

on the block	take it off
on top of	get another
next to	same
under	different

> ...Shall we build with your blocks? Here's a blue one—can you put it on top of the other block? Good. You put it on top of that block. Here's another one. Put it next to the block. Good, you put it next to the blue one. Here's another one. Put this one next to the blue one. Now it's next to the blue one. Can you get another block? You got another block. Put that one on top of the blue one. Let's see—we have all the blue blocks here. They are all the same color. All of these are the same. Can you find a different color? You're right! That yellow is a different color. Can you find another yellow one? Good, those two are the same. Put the yellow block on top of the other yellow block. They are the same color....

Special Considerations

If your child is hearing impaired you can play an auditory training game out of putting them back by covering your mouth with your hand and saying, "Give me a blue block." "Give me a red one" until you have them all back in the bucket.

Kitten In A Keg

This toy is a seemingly simple one with numerous possibilities for effective language play and learning. It consists of several barrels of graduated sizes that fit into each other with the tiniest one containing a little kitten. Each of the barrels is a different color which also helps your child with color recognition and naming.

...Listen, I hear something in the barrel.

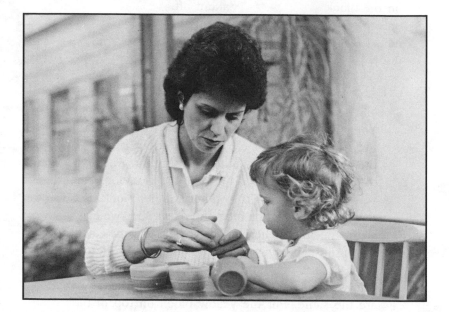

Hand the barrels to your child and help her shake it. If she cannot hear it, she will feel the barrels move inside and you will provide the language that tells her what she feels. If she cannot see it, she will be able to hear and feel the shaking of the barrels.

...I wonder what's inside. Can you guess? (Accept whatever guesses she makes.) Maybe. Let's see if we can find out....

Hand the barrels to your child and tell her to open them up. Most likely she will not be able to do so and you will need to help her. The language you will use involves action verbs such as *twist, turn, pull, open,* and later, *close.*

Single Concept

Let me help you *open* the barrel. I'll twist it. There, it's *open*. *Open* the blue barrel. Can you *open* it? Is it hard to *open?* Good for you. You can *open* the barrel.

Let's open all the barrels. You need to turn the top. Turn it. Can you get it open? Shall I help you turn it? Oh look, there's another barrel inside. Listen, do you hear that? I think there's something else in there. What could it be? Let's open the barrel. Open it. Turn it. Turn the barrel. Well, my goodness, there's another barrel in there. Now we have two. Listen! I hear something else inside. What could it be?

And so on until you arrive at the smallest barrel and say:

...Look at this last wee little barrel. It is so small. Shake it. Well, I don't hear anything. Is there something inside? I don't know. Shall we look? Can you open it? Can you twist the top off? Can you get it open? Oh wow—look at that. There's a tiny little kitten inside. Hi, kitten. Why are you hiding in the barrel? Listen, the kitten is talking. She said, 'meow.' Can you say 'meow' just like the kitten? Oh, the kitten is stuck in the barrel. Maybe she likes it in there. Maybe we should let her go back to sleep. Bye bye kitten. See you later....

Put the smallest lid back on the barrel and twist it to close it while talking about your actions. Then you need to put the other barrels back together again. It is unlikely that your child will be able to size them properly by herself at this age. One way to help her is for you to pick out one part of the barrel and have her find the one that matches it. She will be matching size and color. Continue to find the bottoms of each barrel for her as she finds the matching tops. During this whole process, you can keep reminding her that the kitty is inside and is sound asleep now. As you put the barrels on you may make your voice increasingly softer which will have your child imitating varying intensities. She will need this skill when she is in social situations or school. When her teacher asks her to "lower your voice," she will need to know how to do it.

Another activity that you can do with this toy is to close all of the barrels independently and stack them up from largest to smallest on the top. You can talk about stacking the barrels, putting them *up*, and inevitably watching them tumble *down*.

The language concepts that you will get from this toy are:

color matching   stacking the toy
size comparisons   nesting the toy
hiding concepts   inside of the toy

Fisher-Price House

In the Fisher-Price version of this toy, there are four rooms to the house. There are two bedrooms, a living room, and a kitchen. There is also a garage with a door that goes up and down. Each room has appropriate furniture in it and the garage has a car that

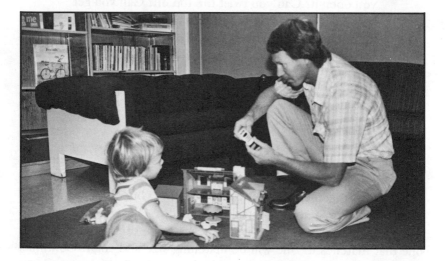

goes inside. With this toy, you can talk about the furniture and the function that each serves. Let's do a play scene with the two bedrooms and then you can create your own play with the other rooms.

There are many ways to play with this toy. The way we've selected is to name furniture. Help your child match each piece of toy furniture with the real furniture in your house.

> ...There are two rooms upstairs. What are they called? That's right, those are the bedrooms. Which one is the room for the little boy (girl)? Okay that looks like the little girl's room. Can you find a bed for the little girl? Good work. Put the bed in her room. That's where she will go when she is tired. What do you do when you are tired? You're right— you go to bed. Shall we put the little girl to bed? Do you think she is tired? Okay, she can stay up and play for a little while. What else goes in her bedroom? I think she needs a bureau (chest of drawers, dresser) to put her clothes in. Do you have a bureau in your room? Let's go and look at your bureau. Which do you think is bigger—your bureau or the little toy bureau? You're right—your bureau is bigger....

Continue in this vein with each piece that you put into the bedroom. Then move on to the parents' bedroom and the other rooms of the house. You will want to name the furniture for your child and have her make the comparisons between the furniture in your house and the furniture in the play house.

Single Concept

This *bed* goes in the *bed*room. It goes right here. Where is your *bed?* Right. It's in your *bed*room. Does Daddy have a *bed?* You're right! Does this *bed* look like Mommy's *bed?* Where shall we put this *bed?* It looks like a very soft *bed*. Do you think it would be a good *bed* to sleep on? Yes, I like your *bed* better too. It is just the right *bed* for a big girl like you.

Once all of the play objects have been labeled and perhaps your child is using words for them, you will be able to create fun play times with the house. Make up stories about the names of the family that lives there. You may want some of your stories to be about things you would like your youngster to do in the house. Perhaps you can talk about the little girl who lives in the play house who picks up all of her toys before she goes to bed at night. If you are having difficulties with bedtime, you may want to plan a play about bedtime activities that the little girl in the toy house likes to do and how she goes to bed on time without a fuss. In the kitchen you can introduce different ways that the play little girl can help her Mom in the kitchen and then provide opportunities for your little gal to help you.

Sometimes there are fears that you can act out during play time. Perhaps you have been going through a fearful time with babysitters and the separation time. You may want to create a play situation that will talk about this fear and get it out in the open.

...Here's the little girl doll. What shall we call her? Okay, that's a pretty name. We'll call her Debra. Here are her Mommy and Daddy. Tonight Debra's Mommy and Daddy are going to a movie. Debra's babysitter will come and stay with her. What is the babysitter's name? Good, let's call her Annie. Here's Annie. Mommy says, 'Debra, Annie's here. It's time for us to leave.' (Now you tell your child) Here, you pretend that you are Debra. What will you say when Annie comes? Why are you crying, Debra? Are you

afraid to stay alone with Annie? Annie says that she
will play a game with you and read you a story before
bedtime. Oh, are you feeling better now? Can you
find a story for Annie to read?...

You don't have to use the real names of your child and the
babysitter but use the names that she wants to use. Do try to imitate what it will be like when the sitter is there. If a boy is the sitter, encourage the use of a boy's name. If you like them to read a
bedtime story, be sure to include that activity in the things that the
sitter will do in the play situation.

Even though your child has an ever increasing receptive
vocabulary you will find yourself doing most of the talking in the
situations where you create the stories. Perhaps you can ask for
input from your child about what to name the characters in the
story. This introduces her to the idea of creative story telling as well
as a vehicle for working out some of her concerns. You may be
surprised one day when you see her playing alone with this toy and
acting out things that she has not shared with you. If you overhear
this kind of play, don't interact then but remember it for the next
time that you have that toy out and encourage the same story she
had created when she was alone.

As we mentioned earlier, any of the toys that represent real
parts of your child's life can be used at any of the age levels interchangeably. The house and objects in it will be fascinating to her
and by the end of this age period, she should know the use of most
items in the house. To help her learn these things, we have included
in this age group, the house set, the tea set, and the toddler kitchen.
All of these, and more, involve items that are common to her
everyday life.

You may want to label some of these items in your own
house. When you make your labels, use upper case and lower case
letters as they are appropriate for the word. You want her to see
them the way they will be seen when she begins to read. Do not
use all capital letters. A great game that your child may enjoy is to
match cards with the names of household furniture and objects to
the actual objects themselves. This early reading readiness should
not be confused with trendy ideas of teaching infants to read. We

suggest this activity just for fun and enjoyment. If you do this activity, tell your child what the word is each time and have her run and match it. You don't want to give her a chance to make an error on this which may affect how she eventually feels about reading. This is simply a fun game that involves written words. If she does happen to learn to recognize a few words from the repetition of the activity, resist showing this skill off to friends and family.

Fisher-Price Toddler Kitchen

The Fisher-Price Toddler Kitchen follows up on her interest in things around the home and particularly the place where families generally spend the most time together–the kitchen. This sturdy set consists of a pan that is also a shape sorter, a milk bottle for filling, a spoon, stacking cups, an oven that opens, a refrigerator that opens, eggs that open up and make a squeaky noise, and various knobs that turn and slide. As you can imagine, there are many ways to play with your child with the toy and many ways that she can play alone.

Let's talk about a play scene that may involve cooking some eggs for breakfast. First you can talk about what to have for breakfast and create the idea that scrambled eggs would be terrific to have for breakfast. You can talk about the fact that eggs come from hens and ask her if she remembers seeing the hens on the farm.

> ...Where are the eggs? Do you want to make scrambled eggs or sunny side up eggs? Okay, let's make scrambled eggs. What do we need? We'll need a pan. Can you find the frying pan? Good for you. Now let's see, we'll need a cup to put the eggs in. That's right, that's a good cup. Okay now, let's see what else do we need? You're right, we need a spoon. Okay we've got a spoon, a cup, a pan. What else do we need? (Laughing) Of course, we almost forgot the eggs. Now we have everything. First we need to crack the eggs into the cup. How many shall we make? Two? One for you and one for me. Okay, crack the egg on the side of the cup.

THE LANGUAGE OF TOYS ◇ 165

That's right; you did it right. Be careful, don't get any shell in the egg cup.

Here's the second one. Crack the second egg. Now they're both in the cup. What shall we do now? Right. We need to stir the eggs. Round and round and round we go—stirring the eggs we go. Okay. I think they're ready now. Put the pan on the stove. Turn it on. Can you turn the dial. Good for you. Put the pan on the stove. Now let's pour the eggs into the pan. Ummmm, that looks good. Stir the eggs in the pan. Cook them all the way through. They look ready now. Shall we sit down and eat them?...

Single Concept

Do you like to *eat* eggs? So do I. We *eat* eggs in the morning. Does Daddy *eat* with us? What does Daddy *eat* for breakfast? It's almost lunch time. Are you hungry? Do you want to *eat* now? What shall we *eat?* Do you want to *eat* a banana?

We'll talk about using a tea set with this age group and this would be a nice time to get the tea set out if your child is still interested in this activity. You can combine making real scrambled eggs and eating them together on her little tea set. When you are cooking with her, which by the way is just a wonderful activity for sharing and learning all kinds of new and exciting vocabulary, be sure and stress safety with her while you are cooking. Remind her never to turn on the stove by herself and never to play near the stove when she is alone. Teach her about hot. Let her feel parts of the stove that get warm enough for her to feel the heat but not hot enough to burn her.

The Tea Set

The kitchen sets that are available at toy stores are incredible. All of the brand names that you might have in your own kitchen are available in the toy department. Our young chefs can have the finest in Pfaltzgraff and Revereware as well as microwave equipment. We really feel you can stop with a tea set. Most of your child's play will involve this tea set and little lunches and breakfasts can be served with them. We would advise you *not* to have your youngster along when you pick out these items as you may end up with more equipment for her than you have for yourself! She will enjoy whatever you provide for her. The tea set gives you an opportunity to teach her the vocabulary for the items that you use for your mealtimes. You can also teach her the correct placement of the items on the table with the fork on the *left* and the knife and spoon on the *right*. Napkin rings for the tea set can be made by decorating a paper towel roll and then slicing it into napkin ring pieces. Your child will enjoy decorating the paper towel roll.

Wonderful table conversations can be created while sitting down to a tea with your child. This might be a time when you can discuss other things that went on during her day. Perhaps you had a

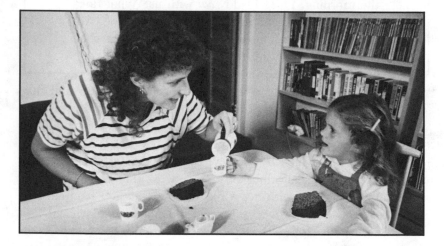

visit to a doctor or a therapist that day and you can chat about it over tea. If at all possible have your tea be something that the two of you have cooked together. Cooking and eating together are wonderful activities for sharing thoughts and feelings.

> ...Yum, these cookies that we made are delicious. Maybe we should save one to give Diane

when we go back on Thursday. This morning when we saw Diane you had to do some interesting jobs for her. Do you remember? You were walking on that straight line right down the middle of the room. You did a good job of staying right on that line. Was that tricky for you to do? No—you thought it was easy. Well, good for you. It looked very tricky to me.

(Child) I liked walking on that line, but I couldn't catch the ball. I'm mad that I couldn't catch the ball.

Catching balls can be tricky. I saw how hard you were trying. Maybe when we get finished with our tea we could play with the ball and you could practice. Then on Thursday, maybe it will be easier for you when you and Diane play ball. Would you like to practice with me?

(Child) Okay, but it is hard for me. Maybe I can't do it.

That's okay. Practicing will be fun. If you can't do it today, maybe tomorrow it will be easier. Remember, you didn't always know how to walk on the straight line but we practiced and practiced and now it's not tricky for you anymore....

Your child may not be able to express all these feelings, but you should be able to keep up a dialogue with her about her feelings of frustration and how you are willing to help her practice. Bringing up successful moments that you observed in the therapy session will help her see that she was successful with some things where others were more difficult.

Cars, Trucks, Road Signs

We have come a long way in our culture where only girls played "cooking" while little boys dug roads and tunnels for their cars and trucks. We encourage you to provide all of these opportunities for your children regardless of their gender.

Matchbox and other companies make very realistic replicas of cars, trucks, and many other vehicles. You can teach unlimited vocabulary with these toys. Each rescue vehicle and construction truck has vocabulary unique to that item. You can teach road safety with toy sets of stop signs, yield signs, and traffic lights.

Setting up roads with blocks and moving vehicles are great activities for your toddlers and her friends as well as terrific teaching time with you. Be sure to use the actual names of the vehicles. For those of us who grew up not knowing a bulldozer from a crane, most of the toy packages are labelled and you can learn them with your child. We have been amazed at how many of the names our children have learned already. Each of these types of cars and trucks have different attributes that you can talk about. The function of the construction truck, the way the doors open on the van, the way the top goes down on the convertible, why there are numbers on the racing car are all good opportunities for introducing language. You can make appropriate vocal noises as you drive the trucks along your highways and squeal the brakes as you stop at the

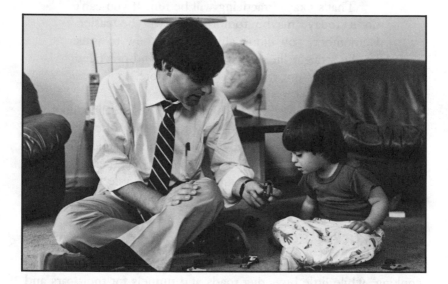

traffic light. As with the house, you may want to make up a story of what the construction people are building and how the different machines help them to do their jobs better and easier. Enjoy yourself and get into the play. If you're a Mom you may find that you get as much pleasure out of these trucks as your child, perhaps because you never had the opportunity to play with them when you were a child yourself.

The large scale version of the Tonka trucks are wonderful for outdoor play in the sand or the dirt. Your child will spend many hours with these large trucks and they are made so well that they will probably last through your grandchildren.

Wind Up Seaplane

Most children by this age really enjoy bath time and can linger in the tub until their fingers look like wrinkled prunes. Although it is tempting to leave your child in the bathtub by herself, thinking that she is playing contentedly and old enough not to get into trouble, we cannot emphasize enough how important it is to stay with your child for safety reasons. She is at a very active and curious stage and at any moment she could decide to climb out of the tub and slip or get into mischief in the bathroom.

Use this bath time together to help develop your child's language. A toy that will help you is Playskool's Wind Up Seaplane. The brightly colored, easy to handle plane, and removable pilot in the cockpit, float. The propeller spins, and the seaplane steadily moves across the water's surface once it is wound up. Your child will be fascinated by all of these features but particularly by the wind-up mechanism and the motion of the seaplane as it drifts around the tub.

Concentrate on providing your child with the language to describe the activity of the pilot and the plane. This is a great time to use your imagination and help your child use hers. Children at this age are developing a real sense of storytelling and fantasy. Ask her questions to stimulate her imagination and use this chance to work on concepts such as *who, what, when,* and *where.*

> ...Where is the seaplane? Who is the man sitting in the plane? You can take him out of his seat. What is his name? Oh! his name is Bill. That's a good name. Now let's put him back in his seat. Put his seat belt on so he'll be safe.

Who does the pilot want to visit in his plane?,
He's going to see his Grandma? What a good idea!...
You can also provide your child with words and phrases to
describe the motion and speed of the plane.

...What can you do to help the pilot start his
plane? That's right. You need to wind up the
propeller. This is the propeller. It's attached to the
plane here. Watch it turn around. Faster...fast-
er...faster. The pilot's really flying now. He's going
straight to Grandma's house. See how the plane
stays on the top of the water? That's called float-
ing. Can you float on top of the water?...

Homemade Toys

My Own Puzzle

A fun activity that you and your child can do together is to make
puzzles. You only need a very few easily found materials including
stiff cardboard. Some sources for this are the cardboard that comes
in shirts when they come from the laundry, old cardboard boxes
that you can cut to size, poster board that you can buy from the
store, and the styrofoam meat trays that you get from the grocery
store. Be sure to wash them carefully so that there are no odors left.

The puzzles that you can make are limited only by your imagination. You can make one from a picture of your child. You can
make it snapshot size or have it blown up into larger size at the
photo store. Mount the picture on the cardboard using a glue such
as Elmer's and then cut the picture into odd shapes. Depending on
the developmental level of your child you can determine how many
pieces to make the puzzle into.

Look through old magazines and find interesting pictures that
you can mount and cut in the same way. For these younger developmental ages, use a picture that is very simple and does not have
more than two or three objects in the picture. You can build up
quite a nice supply of these which you can use for vocabulary building games. If you only cut them into two pieces, you can hold onto
one piece, say the name of the picture, and then have your child

find the other half. You can play a riddle game and hold your half so that your child cannot see the picture half and say:

>...I see a picture of something that is long, yellow, and very good to eat. Can you find the other half? What is that called? You're right—it's a banana.
>Here is part of a banana. Can you find the other half?...

You might want to put a picture on one half of the puzzle and print the word on the other half. This is an activity that is similar to matching the words on the furniture that we talked about earlier. We offer the same caution. Don't expect your child to "read" the words and don't expect her to perform for others if she does happen to learn a few of them.

Making puzzles is a fun activity for you to do with your child and is even more fun when you are playing with them.

Sound Boxes

The idea of this little game is to help your child to listen carefully to differences in sound. You can make as many pairs of sound boxes as you wish. We give you suggestions for items to put in. You can decide which you want to use. Some will be more difficult to hear than others. When you first play this game, use only two different sounds then add one each time you feel your child is ready. If you make this game with your child, she will have the benefit of knowing what kinds of things are inside the containers. To make this game, you will need identical containers for as many sound boxes as you are going to make. We have used film canisters, juice cans, and margarine tubs to make our sound boxes. For our description here, we use juice cans. Carefully clean the juice cans and make sure there are no metal rims to cut your child. We will make ten sound boxes here so you will need ten juice cans all the same size. For the sounds, we suggest rice, small nails, dimes, beans, and buttons. You can use any other items that you can think of. Take the first two juice cans and put the same amount of dry rice into each can. Cover the cans with aluminum foil and set them aside. Continue with the other cans, two at a time filling the two with identical amounts of each item that you use. You can start the game by taking the two pairs of the most different sounds. In our selection, these would be rice and nails.

> ...Listen to this sound. (Shake the can.) This
> is a very soft sound. Listen. Now which of these
> other cans do you think sounds the same?...

Shake each of the other cans in turn. If your child does not correctly identify the matching can, shake them again and you choose the correct one then repeat the above dialogue again.

> ...Good, you chose the right can. Listen again.
> These two sound the same. Now let's see if you
> can find the matching can to this sound....

If this goes fairly easily, add a third set, and so on until she can choose between all five. This is a very tricky listening game. If your child has a lot of difficulty with only two cans, put the game away until later in her development. Do not continue with any activity that is too difficult for your child.

Vocabulary And Concepts

The following list will give you an idea of the vocabulary and concepts that your child should be familiar with.

action verbs (twist, turn, pull, open, close, stir, pour, turn,
   put, wind, float, dance, eat, walk, run, jump)
alphabet letters
babysitter
bottom
child's name, address, and phone number
colors
color matching (same/different)
descriptive words (huge, fuchsia)
directions (left, right)
early reading readiness skills (labeling household objects with
printed words in capital and small letters)
feelings (happy, sad, mad, angry)

first
furniture (bed, chair, sofa, television, table, bookshelf)
garage
get another
hide
hide one inside the other
last
loud
mealtime utensils (spoon, fork, knife, plate, glass, cup, mug)
names of foods (scrambled eggs, fried eggs)
numbers 1-10
occupations (firefighter, painter, pilot, doctor, truck driver,
    teacher, waiter, waitress)
opposites (fast/slow, same/different, first/last, on/off)
please
prepositions (on, under, next to, on top of)
rhymes (Mary Had A Little Lamb)
size comparison (bigger, smaller, same)
soft
sounds cars and trucks make
stack one on top of another
take it off
times of day (morning, night)
thank you
top
traffic signals (stop, go, wait)
truck names (bulldozer, crane, construction truck, mail car-
    rier)
weather (cloudy, rainy, sunny, cool, warm, hot)
what
what's inside
when
where
who
household rooms (bedroom, kitchen, living room, bathroom)

Toy Summary

The following is a list of toys that we have worked with in this developmental year. The * indicates a homemade toy.

cars   road signs
duplo blocks   tea set
Fisher-Price Garage   trucks
Fisher-Price House   Wind Up Seaplane
Fisher-Price Toddler   *puzzles
Kitchen   *sound boxes
Kitten in a Keg
Lego blocks

Books

During this time, your child will begin to be more involved with his books. Bedtime reading should be a ritual by now. Many stories he will have heard so many times that he may be able to *read* them to you. Encourage his participation. Let him tell you the story. You'll be amazed at how accurate he can be. Stories that tell about courage—such as *The Little Engine That Could* and problem solving stories such as *Corduroy* are easy for your youngster to relate to.

ABCing: An Action Alphabet, Janet Beller, New York: Crown Publishing, 1984.

Clear photographs showing kids in action for each of the letters of the alphabet. For example, Dancing, Eating, Jumping.

At Work, Richard Scarry, New York: Golden Press, 1976.

One of a series that focuses on special topics. This one shows various occupations, such as working at home, gardener, tailor, letter carrier, teacher, firefighter, cashier, butcher, baker, carpenter, nurse, dentist, musician, painter, driver, pilot, sailor, airport worker, circus performer. Great opportunity to introduce a wide range of new vocabulary. Other books in this series are:

My House   On the Farm
On Vacation   About Animals

Brown Bear, Brown Bear, What Do You See? Bill Martin, Jr., illustrated by Eric Carle, New York: Holt, 1983.

After several readings of this book, your child will be joining in on the refrains. A few more readings and your child may be "reading" on her own with the help of the pictures and repetitive texts. A favorite with preschoolers.

A cumulative rhyme that begins, "Brown bear, brown bear, what do you see? I see a redbird looking at me. Red bird, red bird, what do you see?"

Corduroy, Dan Freeman, New York: Viking Press, 1968.

An endearing tale that young children have enjoyed for many years. Tells the story of a stuffed bear who searches through the toy store for its lost button, finds a friend and a home.

Great Day For Up, Dr. Seuss, New York: Random House, 1979.

If you ever wanted to focus on a single vocabulary word, this is the book for "up." The catchy and repetitive rhymes make it fun for children to listen to and join in.

Harry the Dirty Dog, Gene Zion, New York: Harper and Row, 1956.

Harry doesn't want to take a bath. He buries his bath brush, runs away, and gets so dirty that when he comes home, no one recognizes him.

I Can, Can You? Peggy Parish, New York: Greenwillow Books, 1980.

This book capitalizes on all of the "I can do it myself" feelings of this age. Gives young children an opportunity to imitate simple actions that are shown in the book that they can do. For example, wiggling fingers, sticking out tongues, and touching their toes. The pictures of children are multiethnic and help any child identify with someone like herself.

I Can Do It Myself, illustrated by June Goldsborough, New York: Golden Books, 1981.

Another example of a book that can help a young child going through the stage of wanting to do everything on her own. This book follows a young child throughout her day and shows all the ways in which she can help around the house and do things on her own.

Is It Hard, Is It Easy? Mary M. Green, illustrated by Len Gettleman, New York: Young/Scott/Wilson-Wesley, 1960.

During this stage of wanting to do things on their own, some children may become frustrated with things they cannot do very well alone. This little book pictures children doing things that are easy and some that are hard. It shows that we all cannot do things equally.

Jesse Bear, What Will You Wear? Nancy White Carlstrom, illustrated by Bruce Degen, New York: Macmillan, 1986.

This charming story is written in verse and takes the reader through the process of getting dressed in the morning and undressed at night. Gives an opportunity to talk about clothes for different times of the day as well as the self-help skills that young children learn at this age.

The Little Engine That Could, Watty Piper, illustrated by George and Doris Houman, New York: Platt and Munk, 1954.

Children enjoy the refrain in this delightful story and get the message that they should continue to try even when they think they can't do the job. This may be especially inspiring for children with special needs who continually need encouragement to try difficult things.

My Very First Book of Numbers, Eric Carle, New York: T. Crowell, 1974.

This is a board book which is spiral bound and cut horizontally so that the child can match the top and bottom halves of the pages. The top has the pictures of a certain number of objects and the bottom has the number.

My Very First Book of Colors, Eric Carle, New York: T. Crowell, 1974.

This book is the same as the number book, except that the concepts being taught are colors. Fine illustrations by this talented artist.

Noisy and Quiet, illustrated by Lorraine Calaora, New York: Grossett and Dunlop, 1976.

The entire book only talks about "noisy" and "quiet" scenes. There are lovely pictures of all kinds of indoor and outdoor scenes with many examples of noisy and quiet on each page. Plenty of opportunity for conversation starters here.

Numbers: A First Counting Book, Robert Allen, New York: Platt and Munk, 1968.

Clearly illustrated book showing the correct number of objects, one concept to a page. There are pages with one kitten, two eggs, three dolls, four pictures, five cars, six buttons, seven flowers, eight candles, nine blocks, ten cookies. An opportunity to talk about numbers and also to name familiar objects.

Push Pull, Empty Full, Tana Hoban, New York: Macmillan, 1972.

Black and white photographs showing opposites. A great "talk about" book for naming as well as to introduce the concept of opposites. The concepts shown are: *push/pull, empty/full, wet/dry, in/out, up/down, thick/thin, whole/broken, front/back, big/little, first/ last, many/few, heavy/light, together/apart, left/right, day/night.*

The Snow, John Burningham, New York: Harper and Row, 1975.

Nice illustrations of all of the fun things there are to do in the snow and then coming indoors and warming up with hot chocolate. A warm book to read while you are curling up with that hot chocolate after playing in the snow.

The Snowy Day, Ezra Jack Keats, New York: Viking Press, 1962.

Another fine book with beautiful illustrations and no text about activities to do in the snow. This one ends with a warm bath after the chilling fun day.

Talkabout Clothes, Ethel Wingfield, illustrated by Harry Wingfield, London: Ladybird Books, 1974.

Talks about all different kinds of clothes for all kinds of weather and people. How we make clothes, colors of clothes, repairing clothing. Opportunities for child to be involved with matching different clothing as well as finding similarities and differences in items of clothing.

The Very Hungry Caterpillar, Eric Carle, New York: Philomel, 1964.

A tiny caterpillar eats her way through different fruits and vegetables on each day of the week for one full week. At the end she emerges as a beautiful butterfly. Concepts here are in the numbers of the things she eats, the days of the week, and the scientific discovery of a caterpillar turning into a butterfly. A classic tale for young children.

The next few pages are checklists for you to evaluate how your child is doing.

SUMMARY OF YOUR CHILD'S THIRD YEAR 24-36 MONTHS

LANGUAGE

Developmental Milestones	Date Achieved	NOT YET	PROGRESSING
uses plurals			
uses noun phrases with articles a an the			
uses three word phrases			
uses possessive nouns which ones?			
uses pronoun "I"			
asks simple questions- who? what? when? where?			
adds "ing" to verbs			
uses past tense for verbs			
uses 4 word sentences			
can say whole name			
can respond to questions with choices			
uses social phrases thank you please			
sings along with music			
outsiders understand his speech			
knows 800 words			

PHYSICAL

Developmental Milestones	Date Achieved	NOT YET	PROGRESSING
Can walk backwards			
can walk up stairs alternating feet holding hands or rail			
can run without falling			
can jump- both feet off floor			
can bounce and catch a large ball			
can pedal a tricycle			
can build a tower of blocks how many?			
can hold crayon not fisted			
can make snips with scissors			
can hold a glass with one hand			
can hold fork in fist			

COGNITIVE

Developmental Milestones	Date Achieved	NOT YET	PROGRESSING
can point to body parts hair tongue teeth hand ears feet head legs arms			
can name body parts mouth eyes nose hair hands ears head			
can match colors orange purple brown black			
can identify colors give me the red car blue yellow green			
can match shapes circle square triangle			

COGNITIVE

Developmental Milestones	Date Achieved	NOT YET	PROGRESSING
can follow directions put the doll in the box put the doll under the box			
can demonstrate knowledge of opposites little big short long			
can demonstrate knowledge of use of common objects What do we do with beds? Why do we have coats?			
develops imaginative play more fully			
able to express feelings			
understands math concept of "just one" Give me *just one* block			

Thirty-Six To Forty-Eight Months

You may be relieved to discover that this can be the "calm after the storm" age. The "terrible twos" has ended and magically your child doesn't seem to have tantrums the way he used to. At the developmental age of three, your youngster has graduated from toddlerhood. He is now quite steady on his feet. And he is much more ready to consider other people's points of view, not just his own. All of these things will happen gradually, not overnight.

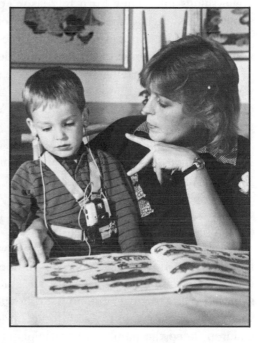

Now he can look at books for quite a long period of time. Since he may be in a transition time with his daytime naps, you may have some bedtime difficulties. This is an excellent time to establish a bedtime routine and books are invaluable for this. We suggest a bath after dinner, followed by a quiet game or toy activity. Then bathroom routines are completed, ending with a story being read by you to your child or he "reads" a book to you. State the number of stories to be read beforehand and then stick to that number. A firm good night with permission to "read" to himself for a few minutes will end your evening with your youngster. Do not be drawn back into the room with pleas of "one more story" or "one more drink of water." Your firmness and consistency are important in order for him to learn limits. Being allowed to "read" for a few minutes gives him the idea that he is in control of when he actually falls asleep. So many of the arguments about bedtime are really "control" kinds of arguments. This compromise solution will avoid many of these arguments.

If your child is not in a preschool program, you might want to consider organizing a play group in your neighborhood so that he can have the opportunity to interact with other children and learn about sharing toys and playing together. You should be within earshot when they are playing together but resist the temptation to step in and solve every problem that comes up. Children need to argue things out. They learn to reason, defend their position, assume leadership, and abandon control through their play at this age.

He will have a better idea of the larger world outside his home and now is when some of his fears may develop. He may be afraid of monsters, or of having you leave him, or of death. Since this is the age when he develops an ability to fantasize, the combination of fantasy and fear can be a potent one. You may have to address some of his fears in your play situations.

Encourage him to share his activities and especially his feelings. You may need to ask questions to spur him on and keep the conversation going. "Then what happened?" "Can you tell me more?" "How did you feel when he said that to you?" Sharing his feelings and his experiences helps him realize that you enjoy listening to him and are eager to discuss things with him.

Now you can begin teaching him how to play games. Waiting for your turn, moving only a certain number of spaces, "reading" the directions, winning and losing are all skills you can teach through games. He'll take great pride in hearing you say, "Mommy likes the way you're sharing your toy with Jodie." If he plays games with other children, keep the number of participants small so that they really have a chance to practice these skills.

Board Games

Typically, board games lend themselves to having a winner and a loser. Instead of emphasizing this aspect of the game, encourage the playing of the game for the fun of it. In this way, winning and losing will take on their proper perspective. Once you have taught your child how to play the games and have used them for your language teaching, he will enjoy playing them with friends. In the begin-

ning it will be helpful for you to be involved in the games to keep
things moving along smoothly.

Candyland

Candyland is a classic and your child will love the bright, sturdy, and colorful board, cards, and playing pieces. Allow your child
to handle the playing pieces freely at first because the game is new
and he will want to touch all of the pieces. As he is doing this, name
all of the playing pieces for him:

> ...See all the bright cards we need for the game.
> There are blue, yellow, red, green, purple, and
> orange. Can you put them all together in a pile?
> Watch me shuffle the cards and mix them all
> together. This is the board that tells us where to go
> when we pick a card. We'll move our little marker
> around the board and match the pictures on the
> cards we pick. Which color marker would you like?
> I'll take red. On your mark, get set, go...pick the
> first card!...

Candyland is a wonderful play opportunity to review colors with
your child or to introduce them if you have not done so already.
Also, you can reinforce the incidental counting that you taught earlier as you two count together the number of squares you must
move. When you play the next game that we discuss, Hi-Ho Cherry-O, you will be teaching more about numbers.

> ...Let's count how many squares you need to
> go before you get to the candy cane: one, two,
> three, four, five...great!...

In addition to teaching colors and counting, Candyland helps
your child practice the social skills of sharing and taking turns. You
may find that he is able to handle sharing and taking turns well when
he is playing with you but will be unable to do this yet with friends.
Help him by playing with him once or twice and if he cannot share

with his friends, then use the game only for teaching times with you.

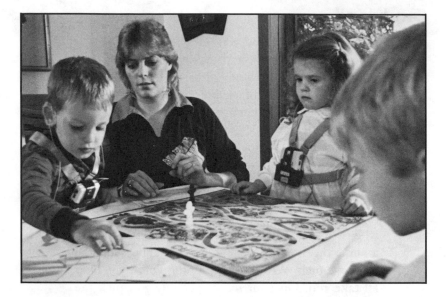

Hi-Ho Cherry-O

This is another classic favorite for this age group. The board for the game has four cherry trees and each one has holes for ten cherries. Next to each tree is a hole for the bucket to fit in. The buckets are red, yellow, green, and blue. The object of the game is to be the first one to pick all the cherries off the tree and fill the bucket.

The spinner has pictures of one, two, three, or four cherries as well as a picture of a spilled bucket. When you spin you can pick the same number of cherries as the number you landed on. When you are first playing this game, you and your child can put the cherries from your tree onto the spinner so that you can actually match the cherries to each other. You can count them out loud as you do it.

...Let's see how many cherries you can pick.
Good. Put one of your cherries on each of the cher-

ries on the spinner. That's one, two, three. You get
to put three cherries in your bucket. Good job....

If you hit the "dump the bucket" then all of your cherries must
go back into the tree. You will enjoy playing this game with your
child and might consider some of the language you can use.

numbers—one to four	take it out
colors—red, green,	pick up the cherry
blue, yellow	cherries
ordinal numbers—	bucket
first, second, third	tree
put it in	

Because these games require only short explanations, they are
excellent for children with language delays. If your child has a visual
impairment, you can put pieces of velcro on the cherries on the
spinner so that he can feel them as he matches his cherries to them.
You may want to put velcro on the little cherries also so that they
can stick to the ones on the spinner and will not roll out of touch
for your child. This will also be helpful if he has physical difficulties and cannot keep all of the pieces from rolling about. With these
modifications, this game will help to promote eye/hand coordination and finger dexterity.

Sesame Street Games For Growing

This set of board games introduces a variety of preschool concepts. Six different game sets can be purchased separately. There
are games that focus on the alphabet, opposites, counting, colors,
shapes, and family/neighborhood members. All of these concepts
are taught using the familiar Sesame Street characters. Each game
comes with a small booklet explaining eight different games con-
tained in each set. We'll look at the game of opposites. The concepts introduced in this game are:

full	day
empty	big
top	little
bottom	under
first	over
last	light
night	heavy

Single Concept

Can you climb to the *top* of the jungle gym? Yes, you can climb to the *top* because you are a good climber. Do you like being at the *top?* It makes you very tall to be at the *top*.

It gets dark at *night*. What do you like to do at *night?* You like your bath at *night?* So do I. I like to eat dinner at *night*. *Night* is a quiet time. You get ready for bed at *night*. Right, we sleep at *night*.

One game is to collect as many of the opposites matching pairs as possible. First you spin and then try and find the card that has the opposite of the picture that your spinner landed on. Be sure to talk about the concepts as you play the game.

> ...Oh, you landed on the picture of 'full.' What is the opposite of full? Hmmm, your glass is *full* of milk. Then you drank it all up. Now your glass is? Right, it is *empty*. Can you find the picture that shows us that it is empty? Shall I help you? That's right, that's the picture that shows empty. You get to keep both cards and now it is my turn....

There are eight different mini games that you can play with these cards. You may even be able to think of new ways to play with them. Perhaps you can ask your child to use the new word in a sentence.

In addition to the opposites, other vocabulary words you can talk about are:

shuffle
spin the spinner
can you match
get rid of all
your cards

pairs of cards
how many pairs do you have?
your turn now
one person at a time

Shape Sorter

There are many varieties of these toys on the market. They range from very simple ones with only three or four shapes to complicated ones such as the one made by Tupperware which has ten different shapes. The pieces are stored inside the ball which can be pulled apart to dump the pieces. Your youngster may find this a little difficult and you may need to help. Also, it may be overwhelming for your child to see so many pieces all at once. Keep them in your lap and introduce them one at a time. Be ready to help your child physically with putting the shapes into the holes once you have found them.

> ...Look, Emily, this shape is called a hexagon. It has six sides. Let's count them. One, two, three, four, five, six. Can you count them now? Good for you. Now where does it fit? Let's look for the hole that has the same shape. Oh, you found it. That's right. Let's fit it in. Wow, you did it. Let's find another shape....

Each of the shapes should be discussed in this way. Use the actual name of the shape and describe what makes it different from other shapes. Your child will enjoy tracing around the edges of the shapes which will give you another opportunity to talk about them.

Single Concept

Let's take the triangle and trace around it. We'll count the *three* sides of the triangle. One, two, *three*. Look, we have a triangle with *three* sides. One, two, *three*. Now trace around the *three* sides and the *three* points of the triangle. Good job.

The Tupperware shape sorter has additional play value in that each piece has a number on the inside. In some cases, it happens to correspond to the number of sides it has but this is not true in every case. You can use the pieces for ordering numbers in sequence from one to ten. For further reinforcement of the number concepts, there are raised dots inside the piece which correspond to the number.

...This shape is a pentagon. It has five sides. Let's count them. One, two, three, four, five. Good. Can you say those numbers? One, two, three, four, five. Now there is also a number five inside. Can you feel it? There are also five dots. Let's count them—one, two, three, four, five. Good counting. Let's see if we can find where the pentagon goes in the ball. Does this hole have five sides? Let's count them. One, two, three. Nope, this isn't where the pentagon goes. The pentagon needs five sides. Let's try this one. One, two, three, four, five. All right! This is where the pentagon goes. You did that very well. Put it in now....

Special Considerations

The raised dots on this toy are a wonderful help if your child is visually impaired. For example, the shape that is a pentagon has five sides and also has the number five inside it. There are five raised dots. You can take your child's finger and have her feel each of the dots while you count them. You can then relate it to the five sides of the shape having her feel them as you count them. When searching for the appropriate space on the ball, you can help her count the sides of the space where the pentagon shape will go.

Wooden Beads For Stringing

Wooden beads are fun at many ages and we find that at this developmental age, your child should have the manual dexterity to manipulate the string and beads well. There are many different bead stringing sets in the toy stores. Your child may also enjoy stringing different types of macaroni and rigatoni that you can dye with food colors.

One bead set, called Threading Beads by Galt Toys, has twenty-five smooth and colorful wooden beads. The lace has a plastic tip on the end which eases the threading process. If you use your homemade beads, you can use yarn and put some scotch or masking tape around one end which will stiffen it enough for it to go through the bead.

Once again, you have the opportunity to talk about colors. The colors in this set are red, blue, green, yellow, and orange. You can ask your child to find a red (or other color) bead and put it on the string. This will test his receptive language or understanding of the color name. You can ask him to choose a bead to put on the string next and then ask him what color it is. This will test his expressive use of the words. Be sure to give him ample time to think of the word. If he doesn't know it say it for him.

There are many ways to play with the beads. You may want to group some by color first before stringing them.

...Let's put all of the blue ones over here. Now let's find all of the yellow ones....

In this way they will be grouped for easy finding when you do the actual stringing.

In stringing you may want to make a pattern with your lace and then ask your child to make one just like yours. You might have one red, one blue, one red, one blue or two yellows, a red, and then a blue. However you want to vary it, matching is a fundamental learning skill that your child will need for many school activities.

...Let's see if you can make a pattern just like mine. I have one red bead, then one blue bead, then another red and another blue. Can you do that? Let me help you. First, let's find a red bead. One that looks just like this. Good, that one is red and it looks just like mine. Okay. Put it on the string. Pull it through. Good for you! Okay, what's the next

color? It's blue. Can you find a blue bead that looks
like mine? That's right. That's a blue one just like
mine. Put it on the string. Pull it through.

Now we have one red and one blue and your
string is beginning to look just like mine. Which
color is next? You're right! The next one is red.
Good thinking. You matched your bead to mine.
Put it on the string and *pulllll* it through. Okay, now
what color is the last one? Right—it's blue. Can you
tell me all of the colors? Red, blue, red, blue. Very
good, now you have a string of beads just like
mine....

Eye/hand coordination is improved by fitting the lace through
the hole and pulling it all the way to the end. In the beginning, you
may want to hold the lace (or the bead) while your child puts the
other through. Sometimes, it is just too difficult for your child to
hold them both at the same time and do the necessary threading.
If this is true for your child, you can help him by holding either the
bead or the string.

...Let me hold the string for you. Okay, now
put the bead over the top of the string. That's
right—you need to get the hole over the string.
Good. Now watch the bead slide right down....

After he places the bead on the top of the string, you move
your hand to hold the top of the string and the bead will slide down.
While it is sliding down you can add speech exercises to your game
by putting the bead through the hole and then saying a long vowel
sound as the bead slides to the bottom of the string. You can vary
the sounds you use such as: ahhhhhh, ooooooooo, eeeeeeeee. Your
child will find this a lot of fun.

Some vocabulary that you can teach with this activity are:

pull it through	here's the lace
through the hole	colors of the blocks

You can talk about the pretty jewelry that your child is making. Is it a beautiful necklace or a lovely bracelet? You will be amazed to see that your child may become interested at a later age in stringing more intricate and delicate beads for making more artistic creations...and the skill began here.

> ...You did a good job of stringing those beads. Let's see how tall a tower you can make. Here's a bead. Put it on top of that one. Up it goes. Here's another one. Be careful. Put it on carefully. You did it! Here's another. Do you think it will fall? Nope, it didn't fall. Let's count how many there are. One, two, three, four. Wow, you put four beads up and they didn't fall. Let's try some more....

Continue until they fall down, which is the highlight of this activity for your child. He may be interested in starting right in again with another tower or he may be finished with this for now. Let his interest level guide you in how much time you spend with this activity.

Most developmental tests for fine motor skills involve counting how many blocks a child can successfully stack up. By this age, he should be able to successfully stack ten blocks.

You can use the beads for counting practice. You can count how many of each color there are. Perhaps you can even get to count all the way to twenty-five although this usually doesn't happen until somewhere around five or older. He should be able to count to three or four by himself. He will be able to give you "one more" and "just one." These beginning math concepts are fun to develop at this age.

Fisher-Price Airport

Your child's imagination will soar when he plays with the miniature people and large airplane that make up the Fisher-Price Airport. He will delight in taking on the role of the passengers (playing himself or Mom or Dad) or perhaps he would like to play the pilot role. He can decide where the plane will go. With this toy, the "sky's the limit" when it comes to learning new language.

With your help, your child can plan and carry out an entire trip to Grandma's house.

> ...Okay, let's pack your suitcase before we get on the plane. Which clothes and toys would you like to pack? You want to take your goldfish, 'Swimmy?' No, he can't go with us! You'll need pajamas, shorts and some shirts. (You can even get into a discussion of weather differences if Grandma lives in a different climate than you.) Now it's time to drive to the airport. Get your money ready to pay the toll on the highway.
>
> Look, there's the airport. See how gigantic it is! It's as high as the clouds. We need to find a parking spot. Be patient. Here we are. This person is called the stewardess. She collects all of the passengers' tickets. Can you give her your ticket? Now let's find our seat. See this little cabin in the front of the plane. That's where the pilot sits. It's called the cockpit. The pilot is the person who flies the plane. Look, he has on headphones....

Once you're into your airplane ride, your child can be the pilot, steward, or passenger. You can then choose another role.

You can talk about loading the luggage onto the trailer which is then loaded into the airplane. You can talk about the meals that are served on the plane.

Best of all you can take a field trip out to the airport even if you're not planning an airplane trip. Sometimes, you can arrange for a pilot to take your child into the cockpit of the plane and show him, all the controls and how the plane goes up and down. Often there are tours of the control towers during quiet parts of the day.

Wet Pets Bathtub Toy

The toy we recommend for this age group is called Wet Pets by Colorforms. Wet Pets are sixteen different spongy animals in bright primary colors which stick to the tub and tiles when wet.

Some of the animals included in the set are a rabbit, goat, dog, whale, kangaroo, alligator, horse, and rooster.

This toy is great for your language delayed youngster because there are so many different concepts that you can introduce including color, grouping according to similarities and differences, serial ordering, and shapes.

Begin by asking your child to put all the same color animals together.

> ...Can you find all the red animals and put them
> on this side of the tub?...

The vocabulary you can review or introduce is practically unlimited. A good place to begin is by reviewing each different type of animal. Start with the more familiar ones like the dog and horse and move into the more exotic ones like the rhinoceros. Once all the animals have been identified with your help, you can discuss the animals themselves.

> ...Isn't that silly that this rabbit is green? Do
> you think a rabbit is really green? No. A rabbit is
> brown, or white, or black or gray....

You can review concepts like *next to, around, above, below,* and *in between.* Once your child has placed the wet animals around the tub, you can ask him:

> ...Which animal did you put next to the tiger?
> Can you put the goat below the kangaroo? Is that
> the dog between the rooster and the rabbit?...

You will probably have to help him with the correct answers, but this is a fun way for your child to learn these language concepts.

Have your child group his spongy critters according to animals that live on the farm, or at the zoo, animals that have a tail, those that have fins, animals that live in the water, or on land, animals that can be pets for children. Let your imagination go, the possibilities are endless.

You could use this toy to talk about shapes. Because the animals are easy to handle and relatively small in size, you could ask your child to arrange them on the wall in the shape of a circle, square, triangle, rectangle, diamond, or oval. Once again, you two will have a lot of fun together while you are strengthening his language skills.

Last, but not least, Wet Pets can be used to introduce the challenging concept of ordinal numbers. Once again, after your child has had a chance to randomly move the wet pets around, ask him to "put them in a line." Then review which animal is first, second, third, and on and on. Have fun!

> ...Can you put the animal you saw first at the zoo on the tub? Was it the rhinoceros? I think you are right. Okay, it will go first. Now what could be second? The dog? All right. That's a good choice. Put the dog second. Why don't we put a yellow animal third? Boy, that's getting to be a great looking parade!...

Homemade Toys

Let's Pretend

This developmental age is when children relish imaginary and dramatic play. "Let's Pretend" gives your child the opportunity to "be like" Mommy, Daddy, his pediatrician, his nursery school teacher, and a variety of other people he comes in contact with.

With their vivid imaginations, three-year-olds do not need elaborate costumes to create dramatic play. Any small props will do such as a travel bag, an apron, scarf, hat, or just about anything you happen to have around the house. For more ideas, see the list of materials at the back of the book.

Through imaginary play, your child can practice and act out his growing understanding of the world around him. He tests his knowledge and ideas about his world by experimenting with what it feels like to be an adult. An added benefit is that acting out a visit to the doctor, dentist, or other health care professional allows your child to work through any fears or anxieties he may have about these situations. This is especially important for the language delayed child who often makes visits to audiologists, speech pathologists, doctors, and other professionals. Acting out visits to the doctor via imaginary play becomes a vehicle through which your child can practice the language he is learning.

Do It Yourself Medical Kit

Our homemade toy in this section, a toy medical kit, stems directly from your three-year-old's growing interest in feelings and fantasy. Actually a good time to introduce a medical kit is right before your child visits the doctor. He may have fears that he can work through this way. If he has a developmental delay that causes him to have to visit doctors or therapists frequently, then this toy may provide a way for him to act out some of the things that will be happening to him.

Some of the items that you can put into this kit are bandaids, gauze, and tape. You can use popsicle sticks for both a tongue depressor and a thermometer. You can mark off temperature lines with a black, nontoxic, felt pen on the "thermometer." Add a red line for the fever reading and you've got it.

A stethoscope is a little more tricky to make. We suggest one way to make one but you can also purchase an excellent working stethoscope from Creative Playthings. It works like the real thing and may be worth the investment as the only thing in the kit that will cost extra money.

To make a stethoscope, you can use an old pair of sunglasses that no longer have the lenses in them. Tie a piece of yarn to the center of the glasses and attach a small dixie cup to the other end. The dixie cup is the part that you listen to the chest with. Do not use any type of medications as part of the kit or substitute candy for pills. We do not want to encourage your child to take or even think about giving medications to other children even if it is pretend. Place all of these things in an old metal or plastic lunchbox to which you attach a big red cross and you have a young doctor-to-be. Now comes the fun part—visiting the doctor!

Your child will inevitably want to take turns role playing a trip to the doctor. Encourage your child's imagination to help dispel his fears and to increase his vocabulary with feeling and action words. Your sample dialogue may go something like this:

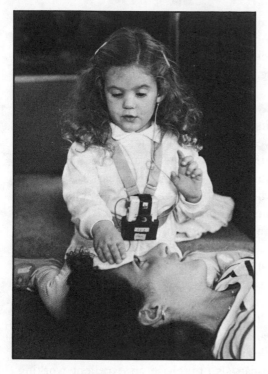

...Would you like to see what's in this medical kit, Cara ? This is a thermometer. We use it to see if you have a fever. You're fine; no fever today. Oooh, look at that scratch on your right knee. We'd better clean your knee with this gauze pad first. There now, that only hurt for a second. Let's put a bandaid on your sore to keep it clean. Very good, you're so brave, Cara....

Now give her a chance to play the doctor role. Perhaps she'll want to try to listen to the patient's chest with a stethoscope. Help her with the vocabulary of the actions she is doing.

...You're going to listen to my chest with the stethoscope. I see. Will it hurt me? No? That's good. I'll sit nice and quietly so you can listen. Are you listening to my heart? What does it sound like? Thumpity, thumpity, thumpity....

Notice in this sample dialogue that much longer sentences can be introduced compared to when your child was younger. He can hold on to more information in his memory and expressively may be speaking in sentences with an average of 5-7 words. He can easily follow the flow of simple adult conversation. Do not be afraid of using technical vocabulary. He will pick it up at his own rate. Using actual words saves you from having to reteach them later on.

Bath Time For Baby

Parents of children this age need to do all they can to promote self-help skills including undressing and bathing. One way to help accomplish this task—and build language skills at the same time—is to encourage your child to wash a baby doll in the bathtub. We recommend any doll of your child's choice, providing it can get completely wet. Some children have a favorite plastic animal that would work just as well. Your child will get so caught up in the fun and excitement of washing his baby doll that he will probably begin washing himself as well. An added benefit is that a great deal of language can be introduced or reviewed in the process.

...Do you want to give your baby a bath tonight? He was playing in the sandbox today and got soooo dirty....

Introduce the concept of undressing for the bath first.

...We need to take your baby's clothes off. First, let's pull the baby's shirt off over his head. Next, let's pull your baby's pants down over his legs. Ooooops, we better take his shoes off first so his pants will slide down over them. Great! Your baby's undressed. He's all ready for the bath. Now, you can get undressed too and you can climb into the bath together....

Once you have talked about the process of getting ready for the bath, you can move on to the next concept of washing the baby doll.

...Let's get all the things you need to wash your baby. Take the soap and hold it with two hands. It's slippery, isn't it? Now take your washcloth and rub the soap onto it. Can you wring out the washcloth? (Demonstrate wringing out the wash-cloth if your child is not familiar with this term.) That's right, you have to squeeze out the extra water. Now you're all ready to wash your baby. First, you can wash your baby's face....

This is a good time to review all the facial parts such as forehead, cheeks, nose, chin, eyes, and ears. Lead your child through a thorough washing of each of these different facial parts on his baby doll, and then move onto the rest of the baby doll's body—arms, hands, fingers, stomach, legs, knees, ankles, feet, and toes. Hope-fully, your child will get caught up again in the excitement and end up washing himself. A simple question from you can get the ball rolling.

...You did such a great job washing your baby. Now can you wash yourself too?...

At the end of bath time, you can talk about drying the baby doll and getting dressed again.

...Your baby doll is getting cold. It's time to get out of the bathtub. (Hopefully your child will get the idea and come climbing out of the tub right along with his doll.) Let's dry off your baby and get your baby's pajamas on. He needs to get ready for bed...and so do you!...

Vocabulary And Concepts

The following list will give you an idea of the vocabulary and concepts your child should be familiar with.

above
action words (shuffle, mix, spin, match)
alphabet
animals (crocodile, alligator, panther)
around

below
beside
body parts (elbows, ankles, knees, shoulders, clavicle)
colors (gray, plum, beige)
counting
doctor equipment (stethoscope, thermometer, blood pressure
    cuff, bandaid, gauze pad)
dress up costumes (apron, scarf, travel bag)
feelings (angry, happy, worried, afraid)
in-between
last night
matching (same, different, bigger, smaller)
negatives (don't, won't, can't)
neighborhood and community helpers (policeman, mailman)
numbers 1-20
occupations (pilot, stewardess)
opposites (full/empty, first/last, day/night, light/heavy)
ordinal numbers (first, second, third, fourth)
parts of animals (tail, fins)
parts of board games (spinner, dice, board, cards, player)
pick it up
pull it through
put it in
rhymes
shapes (rectangle, diamond, oval, hexagon, pentagon)
share
take it out
take turns
today
tomorrow
tonight
use of future tense (he will go)
use of past tense (they went)
use of plurals (children)
why
yesterday

Toy Summary

The following is a list of toys that we have worked with in this developmental year. The * indicates a homemade toy.

Candyland
Fisher-Price Airport
Hi-Ho Cherry-O
Sesame Street Games for Growing
shape sorter
Wet Pets Bathtub toy
wooden beads for stringing
*bath time for baby
*let's pretend
*medical kit

Books

There are many wonderful books which help teach preschoolers such invaluable skills as counting, recognizing shapes and letters, and distinguishing colors. We have two favorite sets of books which should be introduced now. Tana Hoban uses photographs of everyday objects to introduce concepts to children. Some of these are:

Bears in the Night, Stan and Jan Berenstain, New York: Random House, 1971.
A story of the adventures of little bears which uses very few words on each page. The emphasis is on prepositions. The pictures tell more of what is going on in the story than the words do. The prepositions are: in, out, to, at, down, over, under, around, between, through, up.

A series of books that is available through Discovery Toys is called the Ladybird *Box of Books*. The book titles in this series are:
A is for Apple
Colors and Shapes
I Can Count 1,2,3
Nursery Rhymes
Tell Me The Time

All of the books in the Ladybird series are bright and clear with excellent photographs and printed text. Reading these books together will help you teach some of these concepts to your child in a fun and meaningful way.

The Carrot Seed, Ruth Kraus, illustrated by Crockett Johnson, New York: Harper, 1945.

Simple pictures show a little boy's faith in the carrot seed that he plants. No one else believes that it will grow. What a surprise for the grown-ups.

Cat in the Hat, Dr. Seuss. New York: Random House, 1957.

A well-loved favorite for many years. The children's mother goes out on a rainy day. The Cat-in-the-Hat moves in, makes all kinds of messes, but neatly cleans up before Mom walks in the door. A fun story to tell and retell.

Circles, Triangles, and Squares, Tana Hoban, New York: Macmillan, 1974.

An excellent book of photographs of everyday objects that are in the shapes mentioned in the title. Great conversation starter for talking about shapes in our environment and learning to identify them.

Come to the Doctor, Harry, Mary Chalmers, New York: Harper and Row, 1981.

Harry hurts his tail and is scared to go to the doctor, but all ends well for him.

Count and See, Tana Hoban, New York: Macmillan, 1972.

This photographic study of objects focuses on numbers. The numbers one through fifteen are represented and then the numbers are by tens to fifty and from fifty to one hundred. The higher numbers may be too difficult for this age, but this is a good age for exposure to the idea.

Curious George, H.A. Rey, New York: Houghton Mifflin, 1941.

Curious George is like a child in a fur suit. He is always getting into scary situations and being rescued by his protector—the man in the yellow suit. Children enjoy all of the books in the series which involve this little monkey.

Eric Needs Stitches, Barbara Pavis Marino, photographs by Richard
Rudinski, New York: Addison-Wesley Publishing, 1979.
Eric cuts his knee and needs stitches. Medical terms and procedures are clearly explained. Many children will have the experience of needing stitches. This is an excellent book to have on
hand.

Frances Series, Russell Hoban, illustrated by Lillian Hoban, New
York: Harper and Row, 1968.
This series uses Frances, a bear, who experiences many of the
situations that children of this age experience. In *Bedtime for Frances*
we see her posing all of the protests that young children pose when
faced with bedtime. Her parents handle it in a very calm way and
Frances learns. In *Bread and Jam For Frances* we see a typical situation where Frances will only eat what she wants, which happens to
be bread and jam. Her mother and father give her that for every
meal of the day until, of course, she gets sick of it and begins to
see that variety is more fun when it comes to food.
Each of these stories is amusing to young children and also
shows them in a nice way that these problems can be handled and
that other children feel the same way they do.

Going to the Doctor, Fred Rogers, Photographs by Jim Judkis, New
York: Putnam, 1986.
Clear photographs of what children will experience when they
go for a regular check-up. Excellent resource to use before your
child's check-up. Tie this in with the homemade medical kit for this
age and you are on your way to lessening the fear of visiting the
doctor.

Is It Red, Is It Yellow, Is It Blue? Tana Hoban, New York: Greenwillow Books, 1975.
Another excellent photo essay, this time emphasizing colors.
These concept books are an excellent addition to a child's book
shelf.

Madeline Series, Ludwig Bemelmans, New York: Viking Press,
1939.
A classic in children's literature. These lovely stories written in
captivating rhyme have charmed children and adults for many years.
Madeline is one of twelve orphans under the care of Miss Clavell,

and each story tells of the mischief that the smallest one—
Madeline—gets into. A delightful series.

One Fish Two Fish Red Fish Blue Fish, Dr. Seuss, New York: Random House, 1960.

Always a favorite with children, this book emphasizes counting
and color with Dr. Seuss's usual delightful rhythm and rhyme. This
is one you will read and read again many times.

Over, Under, and Through, Tana Hoban, New York: Macmillan,
1973.

A photo essay showing children going through all of these
prepositions. A very nice conversation starter and perhaps an encouragement to have your child imitates these actions.

The Red Balloon, A. Lamorisse, New York: Doubleday, 1978.

No words in this elegant picture story. Tells the story of a lonely little boy who is teased by his friends, but finds a friend in a red
balloon who is always around to help the little boy and take him on
beautiful rides high above Paris. Photographs are excellent.

Rosie's Walk, Pat Hutchins, New York: Macmillan, 1968.

Rosie is totally unaware of the danger when a fox follows her
on her walk. The emphasis is on the prepositions in the story, but
you will not miss the humor of something always happening to the
fox and nothing happening to Rosie. The prepositions included are:
around, under, through, over.

Sesame Street Book of Shapes, Eleanor Feltser, Boston: Little, Brown
and Co., 1970.

Shows shapes in everyday objects, has pages for matching
shapes, finding the ones that are the same and different. Shows how
to make different pictures with shapes. A fun book to follow up with
a cut and paste activity to make some of the pictures shown.

Tale of Peter Rabbit, Beatrix Potter, New York: Warner, 1902.

One of the first books ever to use animals acting like little
children. The story is well known and the drawings are exquisite.
Should be added to your child's personal bookshelf.

Ten Nine Eight, Molly Bang, New York: Greenwillow Books, 1983.

A different slant on counting and a lovely way to say goodnight.
Pictures are charming. Counting backwards from ten little toes to
one big girl who is ready for bed. A sleepy-time favorite.

The Tomorrow Book, Doris Schwerin, illustrated by Karen Gund-
sheimer, New York: Pantheon, 1984.

A very different calendar concept for young children because
their world is largely the "here and now." This simple book shows
that tomorrows begin when you go to bed and talks about all the
new things that tomorrow might bring. In addition to helping to
teach this concept, it is a handy book to have around when the day
is not going well and your child needs to look forward to a new
beginning tomorrow.

Where's Spot? Eric Hill, New York: Putnam Books, 1980.

Finding all of the places where Spot might be hiding gives you
the opportunity to talk about different prepositions: in, under, behind. A delightful book.

William's Doll, Charlotte Zolotow, illustrated by William Pene du
Bois, New York: Harper and Row, 1972.

William loves all of his "boy" toys but he also wants a doll. Finally his grandmother helps to explain to William's parents why he
should have a doll so that he can learn to take care of a baby when
he is a Daddy.

SUMMARY OF YOUR CHILD'S FOURTH YEAR 36-48 MONTHS

LANGUAGE

Developmental Milestones	Date Achieved	NOT YET	PROGRESSING
uses negation don't won't can't			
uses plurals			
asks questions			
can tell of experiences in sequence			
can say age and sex			
uses 5 word sentences			
can deliver a simple message			
can respond to conversation of others			
knows some songs			
knows 1800 words			

PHYSICAL

Developmental Milestones	Date Achieved	NOT YET	PROGRESSING
can walk downstairs alternating feet			
can climb low ladder			
can run smoothly			
can jump several times in a row how many times?			
can hop how many times?			
can catch a large ball bounced by someone else			
can bounce a large ball			
two or three times			
can wind up a toy			
can build a tower of blocks how many?			
can do puzzles of 3-5 pieces			
can put on clothing			
can pull a wagon			

COGNITIVE

Developmental Milestones	Date Achieved	NOT YET	PROGRESSING

can point to body parts
  fingers
  thumb
  toes
  neck
  stomach
  chest
  back
  knee
  chin
  fingernails			

can name body parts
  legs
  arms
  fingers
  thumb
  toes
  neck
  stomach
  chest
  back			

can match colors
  pink
  grey
  white			

can show colors when
  asked
  orange
  purple
  brown
  black			

COGNITIVE

Developmental Milestones	Date Achieved	NOT YET	PROGRESSING

can name colors
  red
  yellow
  green
  blue			

can show shapes when
  asked
  circle
  square
  triangle			

can match shapes
  hexagon
  rectangle
  star			

understand time concepts
  today
  tonight
  last night			

can point to opposites
  tall
  short
  slow
  fast
  over
  under
  far
  near			

can sort objects by color			
can sort objects by shape			
can count to 4			

COGNITIVE

Developmental Milestones	Date Achieved	NOT YET	PROGRESSING
understands ordinal numbers who goes first? whose turn is second?			
can tell about the use of household objects What do we use a stove for? What are dishes for? Why do we need houses?			
Can tell what part of the day is for certain activities When do we eat breakfast? When do we go to sleep?			
plays with friends own age			
can express feelings			
develops more fantasy play			
can match letters			

Forty-Eight To Sixty Months

As you look back over the earlier developmental stages, it is hard to believe how far your infant has come. From total helpless-

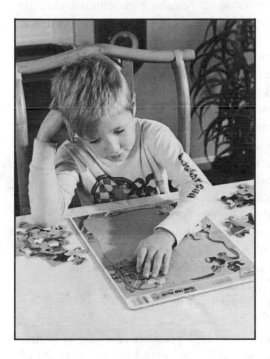

ness, she has emerged as a sturdy individual capable of carrying on long conversations with you. If she has no physical disabilities, she should be able to walk up and down stairs alternating feet on the steps even while carrying things in her hands. She may be able to ride a bike with or without training wheels. She will enjoy coloring and can often draw simple round objects such as balls or apples after you show her how. She will be interested in letters and may be able to trace them and perhaps write

some on her own. We have included some school oriented toys in this category because she will most likely be going to nursery school during this time and may be entering kindergarten. If she has an older brother or sister, she will enjoy doing "homework" while they are doing theirs.

As you have been for the last five years, you are still her model and her teacher. Continue to build her receptive language and give her new and wondrous words for everyday things. She can learn that "huge," "gigantic," and "humongous" are fancy words for big. Children this age just love to play around with multisyllable words. We are sure that their love for dinosaurs at this age is largely because they get to say neat words like "diplodocus" and "tyran-nosaurus rex." Many children are enchanted with the Latin clas-sifications for various types of mushrooms or birds, for instance, and love to talk about them. Continue to talk about all of your daily ac-tivities when you are together. Building an enriched vocabulary will pay major dividends as your child moves along in school and reads and writes. Her knowledge of language will be a valuable asset for her.

While you are continuing to bolster her receptive language skills, you may want to add some idiomatic expressions. Examples of these are "It's raining cats and dogs today;" "My eyes are bigger than my stomach;" "You look as cool as a cucumber." Your child will enjoy learning about these different ways to use and understand words.

Your child will begin to understand time concepts of today, yesterday, and tomorrow. You can help her with this by providing a calendar which is just for her. On that calendar, you can put her regular activities as well as special appointments that are coming up for her. Use pictures so that she can "read" her calendar and you can talk about the time concepts with her.

> "Tomorrow we are going to see Dr. Smith to talk
> about your eyes." "Today Grandma is coming to
> have lunch with us. What shall we make?"

We do not recommend a lot of high pressure teaching at home, but you can begin getting your child interested in school types of activities. Having lots of paper, crayons, and other art materials around will help her develop the fine motor skills for beginning writ-ing next year. Coloring books help with learning how to stay within lines. Balance this with plenty of large paper that she can color within or without lines. Our favorite source of coloring paper is a huge roll of white shelf paper from the grocery store. It is inexpen-sive and lends itself to borderless pictures which can become wall murals or a painting that can be added to over a period of time.

Your play with her can include some basic concepts of num-bers, letters, and prepositions which will be fun for her to learn. Resist having her "recite" her letters and numbers for friends and family. She doesn't need the stress of performing at this age.

Fisher-Price Play Desk

This is a very compact little toy that your youngster can tote around with her from place to place. Many parents have found it invaluable for keeping their children occupied while waiting in doctors' offices. It has a tray which holds plastic letters, a chalkboard and chalk, and a storage place for the word cards which come with it. You can encourage her knowledge of the letters of the alphabet by placing them in the tray in order. This is a lot of fun when you sing the letters in the alphabet song as she hands them to you. You can slow the pace of your singing to match her ability to hand you the correct letters. If you are teaching her the letters and she doesn't know them yet, put them in order as you sing the song. Several rounds of this and she'll begin to add in a few as you go along. Keep offering her opportunities to choose the right one as you go along. She may know "p" when she didn't know "a" or "b."

The word cards that come with this set are of objects that are familiar to your child. There is a picture on the card and then spaces where the letters can fit in. Each space is in the shape of the letter that belongs there. This is an excellent way for her to learn to recognize the letters. When you choose a card, ask your child what the picture is. Let's say that the one we're talking about now is the picture of the *tree*. Your child will know the name of the picture. Now ask her if she can think how the word "tree" begins. Help her listen as she sounds out the word. Give her the opportunity to guess twice and then tell her.

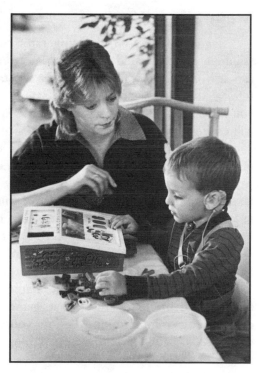

If she has not guessed it by the second try then she really doesn't know and may get frustrated by the game. If she is able to sound out the beginning letter, ask her if can find the plastic letter that shows that sound. If she correctly picks out the "t," help her place it in the correct space on the picture card and then move on to the next sound in the word. If she has successfully placed all of the letters even with your help, be lavish in your praise as this really is an accomplishment at this young age.

Depending on her attention span at this point, you can continue with other cards or show her how she can use the card to trace the letters in the spaces. The picture card fits into a slot at the bottom of the chalk board. She can trace the letters and she can also copy the letters above the letters in the picture card.

The idea here is not to teach your child spelling, reading, and sounding out letters, but to give her the opportunity to play with the letters in a fun way. If it comes naturally to her and she enjoys it, then she will continue to see letters and reading in a fun way.

Magnetic Letters

Magnetic letters on the refrigerator can provide a lot of entertainment for your child as well as more teaching time for you. You can ask her to tell you the letters as she takes them on and off the refrigerator. You can play a game where she asks you a word and you tell her the letters that she needs to spell that word. Your child will especially enjoy spelling the names of members of your family and her very own name! Avoid problems and buy two or more sets of letters so there will be enough letters for those indispensable words with double letters such as "Daddy" and "Mommy." You can be sure that these will be on the list of things that she is interested in learning to spell. She may want to use her card from her Fisher-Price Play Desk to help her spell out words on the refrigerator.

When she is ready, you can add to your game the difference between the names of the letters and the sounds that they make. For example the letter "b" says its name of "bee" but has a sound of "buh." Or the letter "m" says its name of "em" but has a sound of humming–mmmmmmm. Follow your child's lead and give her what she is ready for and interested in.

What word would you like to spell with your
letters?
(Child) Dog.
Okay. Listen while I say the word 'dog.' What
sound do you hear first?
(Child) "Bee."
Listen again. 'Dog.' The first letter is 'Dee' and
it sounds like 'Duh.' Can you find the 'Dee' letter?
(Child holding up the "D" letter) Is this one
'Dee?'
That's right. That's the letter 'Dee.' Do you
remember how it sounds?
(Child) Duh.
Good job! You did a fine job of listening.

Continue with all the letters for the word "dog." Help your child
with the sounds and with finding the letters. This activity should
be fun and not stressful. Remember that you are playing and not
actually "teaching" her the alphabet. She will be able to learn them
better if you make it fun for her.

Dominoes

Dominoes can be played from a very simple matching level to
very complicated levels. Of course, we suggest the matching level
at this time. There are many types of picture dominoes as well as
number dominoes available. We'll tell you a little about each and
how they expand into other matching activities for learning purposes.

The picture matching sets are usually made of cardboard and
have a picture of a familiar object or animal on either end of the
rectangular piece. The simplest form of play is to have all of the
pieces remain face down in a pile; you and your child each take
turns picking one to see if it matches either end of the piece(s) that
are face-up on the table. Dominoes is an excellent game for learning to take turns as well as to observe. With the pictures you have
lots of opportunity to talk about what is represented. Talk about
the color, size, and use of the object. If it is an animal domino, talk
about the characteristics of the animals pictured—how they look,

what they eat, how they make sounds. This is another opportunity to remind her of her visit to the zoo, the farm, or whatever excursion is appropriate here.

...We're going to play with the dominoes now. Can you help me turn all of the dominoes over? These dominoes have pictures of animals on them. Can you tell me their names as we turn them over? Good, you know a lot of animal names. Okay. You can go first and pick one of the dominoes. Let's see. That one has a horse at one end and a duck at the other. I'm going to choose a domino from the pile and see if it matches the horse or the duck. I picked a sheep. It doesn't match the horse or the duck. I'll have to pick another domino. Oh, good, I got one that has a horse on one side and a fish on the other. I can match the horses.

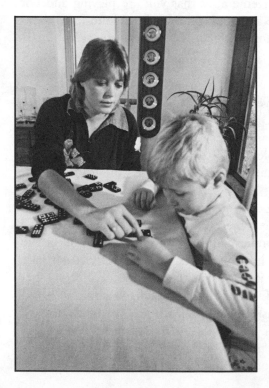

Now it's your turn and you need to find either a duck or a fish. Do you know that both a duck and a fish can swim in the water? The duck uses its feet to swim and the fish uses its fins. Can you see the fins on the fish? That's right. Those are the fins....

If you are ready to move into simple counting you can "deal" out a certain number of dominoes to begin the game. For example, start with three each and count aloud deliberately as you "deal" out the pieces. If you think she is ready, have your child imitate the counting with you. If she is able to count to three alone then give her a turn to be the "dealer."

Single Concept

Let me deal the dominoes. Here are *three* for you. *One, two, three*. Now I'll deal *three* dominoes for myself. *One, two, three*. Can you count with me? *One, two, three*. Great, you counted *one, two, three* with me.

If your child is taking an interest in counting and you feel she is ready, you can use the dominoes that have the dots on them. The numbers only go up to six so it is an excellent beginning counting game. Some of the number sets are also color coded so that each piece that has one dot on it is red, whereas six dots may be yellow. This gives your child an additional way to recognize the piece that she needs to add to the dominoes.

When you begin counting, have your child put her finger on each dot as she says the number. If she is not ready for counting herself, you can take her finger and point to each dot as you say the number names.

It may be difficult at first to explain the idea that the first one who uses up all of her tiles is the winner so you may want to play until the pile is used up and then see who has fewer pieces left. The concepts of *fewer, less,* and *more* are some of the very early concepts that your child will need when she starts school. This is an excellent game for teaching those concepts. You don't have to wait until the end of the game to teach them. As each piece is put down, you can ask about the two numbers on the piece. Which number is more and which is less. Keep varying the way in which you ask her so it doesn't turn into a boring exercise in counting.

As with all of the language that you have taught so far, she will understand the concepts before she is able to accurately express them. Your job is just to keep putting the information in.

Scrabble Alphabet Game

This game is excellent for matching letters to words. It involves the same concepts of taking turns, waiting for your turn, winning and losing, as well as matching letters to words. It helps prekindergarten children recognize letters, and the sounds they make. The way this game is structured makes learning natural and enjoyable.

The letters of the alphabet are on the board and as you move your marker about the board, you can choose the letters that you need to complete the word card that you have. One side of the card has pictures with the words while the other side only has the word. It teaches matching letter to letter as well as the idea of individual letters making up the word.

The letter pieces in this game are made of plastic and can be used for tracing which gives eye/hand coordination practice which your child will need in order to learn to write. If your child can say the letters as she writes them, she will be using many senses at once.

The word cards of this game can also be used for a concentration type game. You can turn three or four cards over, word side down. Then you can spell out the word and have your child find the correct one. If using four cards is too difficult, start off with only two.

Single Concept

Here are two cards. Can you find the letters that go on this card? I'm going to spell a word...C A R. That spells car. You spelled it right. Good for you! You can also use the word cards for riddles.

I am thinking of a word that starts with 'T' and has many branches. Can you find the right card? Good for you, you found the word that starts with 'T' and has many branches. It is the word 'tree.' Now you ask me for a word.

You can take turns with these games so that she has her chance to be the leader. Keep the game fun and she will enjoy it for many months to come.

Mattel See 'N Say For Safety

There are never enough ways to teach your child to be wary of strangers and when to say "no." This toy is a fun way to learn some safety rules and is very appropriate to this age group. You will want to use this toy with your child because you have to be careful to fully turn the pointer and to pull the string all of the way out to get an accurate recording of the message. Some of the safety messages on this toy are:

1. I never cross the street alone. I always hold a grownup's hand.

2. I'm nice to my friends when we play, I never push or shove.

3. I let grownups do the cooking, I never touch the stove.

4. We stay away from fire. It's dangerous.

5. I never talk to strangers. I only talk to people I know.

6. We pick up our toys off the floor, so we won't trip and fall.

7. I only eat what my parents give me—nothing else goes in my mouth.

8. I'm careful in the bathroom. I don't want to slip or fall.

9. Knives and tools are dangerous. I never touch them.

Quarreling among friends is not unusual among young children. One of the rules on this toy is "I'm nice to my friends when we play. I never push or shove." When you are playing with this toy with your child, you might want to discuss an incident that happened. For example:

...Do you remember what happened this morning when Eric wanted to play with your wagon?

> What did you do? That's right. You shoved him.
> What do you think you could have said to Eric?
> That's a good idea. You could have said, 'Eric, I'm
> not finished playing with the wagon yet. Can you
> wait a minute?' Listen to what it says on our safety
> toy. Listen. The little girl on the toy said, 'I'm nice
> to my friends when we play. I never push or shove.'
> Do you think you can try this tomorrow when Eric
> comes over? I'm sure you can....

These are common family rules, and using this toy as a tool makes learning them fun and also somewhat less like another set of orders from you. Your child may think it is more fun to hear from this toy that she should pick up her toys than it is to always hear it from you. You can, in turn, use it as a tool. You can say, "Remember what the Safety See 'N Say says about picking up your toys."

Art Material Toys For The Bath

There are several kinds of art materials designed to enhance your child's pleasure in the bathtub. We think these toys are great for language development for a couple of reasons. One, artistic materials lend themselves to creative free expression that can be used as a basis for language dialogues. Children at this age in particular have vivid imaginations which you can encourage and stimulate by providing the right materials and asking the right questions.

Another reason is that your child's fine motor control has improved greatly from the previous developmental age. She now can take a great deal of time to work on an artistic masterpiece and will feel a great sense of pride on its completion.

There are many fine bathroom toys available. One is Scribble Stix by Coleco and another is Funny Color Foam from Creative Aerosol Corporation. Most of these toys are designed specifically to be used in the bathtub. This means they will not stain your tub or tiles, or your child either! They come in a variety of bright primary colors. Also, because a mild, nontoxic soap is an ingredient in each of these toys, your child can use these materials to create bubbles, and to wash herself.

We recommend that with any of these toys you let your child create the ideas for the pictures and designs. Rather than asking, "Julie, can you make a happy face?" ask "Julie, what can you think of to make?" If she draws a blank, which happens to even the finest artists from time to time, then offer a few ideas. Once she begins to draw, paint, or produce a molded foamy shape, begin to stimulate her imagination even further.

> ...Julie, what will you make today? A puppy...what a good idea. What color will you make him? I see your puppy has ears, legs, and a tail. How many ears? How many legs? Where does your puppy live? At your house? Can you draw a picture of yourself next to your puppy?...

If your child is not ready to create pictures, encourage her to experiment with the basic properties of each of the materials and create designs.

> ...The foam is bouncy. If you make a little ball, it will stick together. Look how it floats on the water. Can you paint a long line? Now can you make short, little dots? Great. Now, how about putting two tiny circles on the inside? That will be the eyes. Can you make a nose? What about a mouth? Look, you made a face. That's great. You can wash it all away and make something else if you want....

No matter what your child's disability is, or the nature and extent of her language delay, these art material toys can be enjoyed greatly and can help her with her language skills. Just let your child's imagination be your guide.

Let's Make Music

We have not talked very much about music with your child. You can include it from the very beginning of your child's life through lullabies and baby songs that lull her into a peaceful sleep. You can keep music on during the day. Perhaps you like classical music,

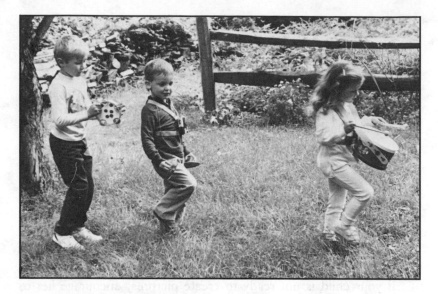

show music, or pop music. Whatever brings you pleasure will bring her pleasure. There are many records that are available for children. Singing with her, doing finger plays such as "Eency Weency Spider," to songs and just dancing about the room with her are marvelous fun activities.

We suggest musical instruments at this level that your child can make with you. If you want them around at earlier ages then you can make them and just have your child join you in playing with them. At this age, however, she can be an active participant in making them.

Drum

Any pot will do with a wooden hammer or spoon for a drumstick. Give her an old pot that she can keep for this purpose. Another type of drum can be made from an oatmeal cylinder container. If you take both ends off the container and stretch some thin rubber such as a balloon across the top, you will have a drum. Once again, a wooden spoon can be used for the stick. Different sounds can be made by different sizes of containers.

Single Concept

Let me hear you *beat* the drum. Take your stick
and *beat* the drum. Boom, boom. *Beat* the drum.
Can you *beat* the drum fast? Now, can you *beat* the
drum slowly? Can you *beat* the drum loud? Now,
beat it softly. Very good.

Castanets

Juice cans make great castanets. After they are opened, cleaned,
and dried carefully, put in some beans or rice. Seal the top very
thoroughly with paper and tape. Shaking the cans will produce different sounds depending on what you put in them. Rice will make
a very soft sound while beans will be much louder.

Single Concept

Shake your castanets. *Shake, shake*. Listen to the
pretty sound when you *shake* your castanets. Can
you *shake* them loudly...hard...slowly...fast?

Rhythm Sticks

Any two wooden objects that can be banged together can be
used as rhythm sticks. You can purchase dowels at a hardware store
or use your old faithful wooden spoons.

Single Concept

Hold a *stick* in each hand. That's right. One *stick*
in your left hand and one *stick* in your right hand.
Now beat the *sticks*. Rat, rat, rat. Good. Can you
beat the *sticks* fast...hard...slowly...soft? What great
rhythm!

Tambourine

Use two aluminum pie pans. Fill one with metal bottle caps. Put
one pan on top of the other to make a container. Punch holes around
the edges with a pointed scissors and then string them together.
You and your child will enjoy doing this project together but be safe

and do the hole punching yourself. The sound that this will make when tapped will be similar to a tambourine.

Single Concept

Listen to what happens when you shake your tambourine. *Listen* carefully. It is very soft now. I am *listening* too. Can you shake it hard? *Listen* to that! Boy, is that loud. It is easy to *listen* to loud sounds.

Bells

Bells of different pitches can be purchased in a craft store. You can sew the bells to a piece of leather or other material. Your child can shake the bells in rhythm to music.

Single Concept

Let's listen to the *music*. Listen, the *music* is very soft now. Can you shake your bells softly with the *music?* Ooops, the *music* stopped. Listen. It's very quiet. When we hear the *music* you can shake your bells again. Your *music* is good to listen to. I like it. Can you shake your bells hard? The *music* is very loud. Great job. You made *music* with your bells.

We're sure you can think of other musical instruments that you can make with your child. When you play with her, you will be teaching her listening skills. If you play a record, have her play along but when the music stops, she must stop also. This is difficult for small children because they so enjoy making the music, but it is an excellent listening skill for them to learn to develop. When you are first teaching her this skill, you will want to start with her seated on the floor with you, watching as you turn the music on and off. If she is sitting near you on the floor, you can reach out and stop her hand from making the sound.

After she has the idea of the activity and is able to stop making music when the music stops, you can get up and move about the room marching while playing the musical instruments. You can add galloping and skipping to the rhythm of different music.

When you are teaching her this listening activity, your conversation might sound like this:

> ...I'm going to turn the record on now. I want you to keep your bells quiet until I turn the music on. When the music stops, then you stop playing your bells. Okay. Here's the music. Good—you're playing your bells. You can make pretty music too. Watch, now I'm turning the record off. Stop playing your bells. Good job—you stopped when the music stopped....

If she doesn't get the idea at this point, you can hold her hand and stop the bells and tell her that the music has stopped and the bells have to stop too. Then try it again. Most children catch on quickly to this idea.

Public libraries often have excellent record collections for young children. Ask your librarian about them. Having a source such as this makes it possible to vary the types of music your children listens to.

There are excellent musical stories on records that you can listen to with your child. Often there are story books that you can get to go along with the listening activity. In some areas there are "lollipop" concerts which introduce children to classical music early in their lives.

Special Considerations

Listening to and appreciating music is a marvelous activity to share with your child. If she has a hearing impairment, do not automatically deprive her of the fun of music. We are never quite sure exactly what sound is like for a hearing impaired child, so go ahead and expose her to the activity. Begin with music that has actions to go along with it or finger plays and you may be pleasantly surprised to see how much enjoyment she gets from this activity.

Playing Cards

Playing with cards is an activity that your child will enjoy doing with you. They are a wonderful source of activities for counting, sorting, and putting numbers in order. You can either buy a deck of cards or you can make them. If you decide to make them, cut fifty-two pieces of cardboard the same size as playing cards are. Then you can color them according to the suits and numbers.

> ...Here's a deck of cards. Can you help me find all the red hearts? Let's put all the red hearts in this pile over here. Okay, now let's find all the red diamonds. This shape is called a diamond. Can you find all the red diamonds? Okay. Now we have a pile of red hearts and a pile of red diamonds. How about this one now? This is a black spade. We can find all the black spades. Put them in a pile over there. Now all the rest are black clubs. What is this shape called? It is a club. Can we put all the hearts in the right order? What comes first? This one with the "A" on it is called an ace and it is the same as number one. So the ace is first. Now can you find the two? Good, that's the number two. See. There are two hearts and the number two. That comes after the ace which is the number one. Now can we find the next one? What comes after two?...

Continue through all the numbers and face cards for each of the suits. This will give your child lots of practice in counting either by imitating you or actually counting the correct number of hearts, clubs, diamonds, or spades. Children will enjoy learning the names and values of the face cards as well.

There are many card games that children of this age enjoy. The one most trying to your patience is the seemingly never-ending game of "war." You may want to set a time limit for this game rather than a winner. To play, divide the deck in half. Each of you places the top card from your pile face up in front of you. The card with the higher value is the winner. This is excellent for helping your child with the concept of "more" or "less." This is one of the basic concepts that kindergartners should know by the end of the school year.

> ...This game is called 'war' because one of our cards will win over the other. You put down your top card. You have a five and I have a four. Which one is more? Is five more than four? Yes, five is more than four so your card is the winner....

As the numbers get higher, you may have to help your child with knowing which is more or less. If this is too difficult, you can sort the deck and use only the lower numbers. This will also shorten your game time. Add in the higher numbers one at a time until she is comfortable with all of them.

Vocabulary And Concepts

The following list will give you an idea of the vocabulary and concepts that your child should be familiar with.

above
adjectives (huge, gigantic, tiny, humongous)
art materials (markers, pastels, tissue paper, construction paper)
behind
below
beside
by the
children's songs
counting 1-20
dinosaur names (diplodocus, tyrannosaurus rex)
fairy tales
feelings
fewer
higher
idioms (It's raining cats and dogs.)
in front of
last week
less
letters of the alphabet

lower
more
musical instruments (castanets, drum, rhythm sticks, tam-
    bourine)
nursery rhymes
opposites
safety rules (never talk to strangers, children don't touch
    matches, look both ways before crossing the street)
ships and boats
sounds of letters
spelling of words
telling time (big hand, little hand)
things in space (stars, planets)
tomorrow
transportation vehicles (cement truck, dump truck, steam
    shovel, jeep, taxi, race car)

Toy Summary

The following is a list of toys that we have worked with in this
developmental period. The * indicates a homemade toy.
    Scribble Stix
    Funny Color Foam
    dominoes
    Fisher-Price Play Desk
    magnetic letters
    Mattel See 'N Say for Safety
    Scrabble Alphabet Game
    *playing cards
    *musical instruments

Books

Books which focus on special interest areas are fun for this age
child. They are interested in a variety of topics and can get heavi-
ly into books about dinosaurs, rocks, or trucks.

Airport, Byron Barton, New York: T. Crowell, 1982.

Clear, beautiful pictures tell what happens on an airplane trip from arriving at the airport to the take-off of the plane. A great prelude or follow up to an actual visit.

Big Truck Book, Janet and Alex D'Amoto, New York: Renewal Products, Inc. 1968.

A board book which shows the following kinds of trucks: farm truck, moving van, gas tanker, delivery truck, cement mixer, steam shovel, dump truck, milk truck, mail truck, car carrier, sanitation truck, ice cream truck. Great for vocabulary and discussion.

The Car Book, William Dugan, Wisconsin: Golden Press, 1968.

All different kinds of cars are pictured here. Big cars, little cars, police cars, campers, homemade racers, ambulance, fire chief car, taxi, jeep, sports car. Great for vocabulary and discussion.

Dinosaur Days, David C. Knight, illustrated by Joel Schick, New York: McGraw Hill, 1977.

Many children at this age are into these prehistoric monsters. This book has simplified drawings with a general description of dinosaurs and the times they lived in. Fun to practice saying those incredibly long names.

Each Peach Each Pear Each Plum, New York: Viking Press, 1978.

Familiar nursery figures such as Jack and Jill and Mother Hubbard are hidden in the pages of this book. The rhyming words continue from page to page. A fun book for learning to look for clues and details.

Everyone Knows What A Dragon Looks Like, Jay Williams, illustrated by Marcos Mayer, Japan: Four Winds, 1976.

Fire, Fire, Gail Gibbons, New York: T. Crowell, 1984.

A nice book to precede and follow a trip to the fire station. Talks about how firemen handle fires in the city, country, forest, and waterfront. Lots of new vocabulary and opportunities for discussion about fire as a safety issue.

The Freight Train Book, Jack Pierce, New York: Carol Rhoda Books, 1980.

Black and white photographs show locomotives, boxcars, tank cars, auto carriers, hoppers, flatcars, refrigerator cars, and cabooses.

Good for vocabulary building and discussions. Take a trip to a train museum or freight yard to see the real things.

Harbor, Donald Crews, New York: Greenwillow Books, 1982.
Colorful pictures of activities in and around a harbor with different kinds of ships and boats.

Leo The Late Bloomer, Robert Kraus, illustrated by Jose Aruego, New York: Windmill Press, 1971.
Leo, a tiger, is slow to talk, read, write, and draw but when he is ready, he does learn. Another example of a little child in animal's clothing. An excellent story for a special needs child who may be a little slower than her friends in learning new things.

Little Toot, Hardie Gramatky, New York: Putnam Books, 1939.
A classic tale of a playful tugboat who didn't like to work until he was faced with a dangerous situation.

Mike Mulligan and his Steam Shovel, Virginia Lee Burton, New York: Houghton Mifflin, 1939.
Another story similar to *The Little Engine That Could*, and *Little Toot*, of a smaller and less able steam shovel beating the more modern fancy equipment. An excellent example for special needs children who may have to work a little harder to achieve their best.

Rain, Peter Spier, New York: Doubleday, 1982.
No words in this lovely story of two children exploring the rain.

Swimmy, Leo Lionni, New York, Pantheon, 1968.
A story with beautiful pictures that tell a tale of a little fish who is different from the others. He is the one to save his friends in the story. Nice for special needs children who may feel different from their friends.

The Truck and Bus Book, William Dugan, Wisconsin: Golden Press, 1972.
This is a paper shape book with pictures of a tank truck, moving van, dump truck, mail truck, coal truck, garbage truck, telephone truck, cattle truck, tow truck, fire truck, school bus, motor bus for trips, and ice cream truck. Good for vocabulary and discussion.

The True Book of the Mars Landing, Leila Boyle Gemme, New York: Children's Press, 1977.
Full page illustrations and photos of the planet Mars. Photos were taken by the spacecrafts, Mariner and Viking. There is a clear and simple text for youngsters who are interested in space.

The Shopping Basket, John Burningham, New York: Thomas Crowell, 1980.
Tells the story of a young boy going to the store to buy six eggs, five bananas, four apples, three oranges, two donuts, and a package of potato chips. Counting and naming as well as preparation for trying out a shopping list with your child when you go to the store.

A Special Trade, Sally Wittman, illustrated by Karen Guntersteiner, New York: Harper and Row, 1978.
A special book for special needs children. Old Bartholomew pushed Nelly in her stroller when she was a little girl. As time passes and old Bartholomew needs a wheelchair, Nelly is happy to push him. A very special book.

The Story About Ping, Marjorie Flack, New York: Penguin Books, 1977.
The little duck, Ping, does not hear the call from Mother to come home and when he finally realizes it, everyone else has left. Afraid of being spanked, he hides and ends up in many frightening adventures. After being caught and almost cooked for dinner, he is set free and finds his way home again, happy to be safe and secure.

Whistle for Willie, Ezra Jack Keats, New York: Young Readers Press, Inc., 1970
. This little boy wants to learn to whistle very badly. He tries many ways and many times and finally does learn. A nice story about sticking to something until you can do it. Important for special needs children who face this every day.

The following books can be used for "problem solving" discussions with your child.

A Birthday For Frances, Russell Hoban, New York: Harper and Row,
1968.

One of the hardest things for young children is to *not* be the
Birthday person. Each child will have a day like that during the year.
This book helps a young child to understand those feelings.

*My Mama Says There Aren't Any Zombies, Ghosts, Vampires, Creatures,
Demons, Monsters, Fiends, Goblins, or Things*, by Judith Viorst

Explores some of the fears of night creatures that some children
have.

My Mother is Lost, Bernice Myers

Talks about what happens when a little boy gets lost in a department store.

When I Have A Little Girl, Charlotte Zolotow, New York: Harper
and Row, 1965.

It is difficult to understand why there have to be so many rules
when you are young. This book helps with those feelings.

Conclusion

We have traveled along an interesting journey from the first
sound of the birth cry to complicated thoughts of diplodoci and
fungi. Your patterns of communication with your child should last
throughout your lifetime together. You may be amazed that your
teenager will share her thoughts with you because she knows that
you have always been there to listen to her. In teaching her language skills, you have not only opened up a world of communication, but helped her gain the confidence she needs in order to
participate fully in the adult world. Because your child has special
needs for learning language, this road to language development may
be challenging for you, but spending time with her now giving her
the gift of language will bring rewards later.

Summary Of Your Child's Fifth Year 48-60 Months

Language

Developmental Milestones	Date Achieved	NOT YET	PROGRESSING
asks for definition of words			
can define more common words and tell how used book, shoe, table			
almost complete use of correct grammar			
uses 6-8 word sentences			
knows the names of siblings			
knows town or city			
knows street address			
uses social phrases excuse me			
can carry on a conversation			

PHYSICAL

Developmental Milestones	Date Achieved	NOT YET	PROGRESSING
can walk down stairs carrying object			
can skip alternating feet			
can do a broad jump how far?			
can hop how far?			
can throw a ball how far?			
can play rhythm instruments in time to music			
can ride small bike with training wheels			
can do puzzles that are not single pieces how many pieces?			
can hold a pencil in proper position			
can color within lines			
can cut with scissors			
can use knife for spreading			

COGNITIVE

Developmental Milestones	Date Achieved	NOT YET	PROGRESSING
can identify all body parts			
can name all body parts			
can name all colors			
can name all shapes			
understands directions using prepositions by the beside below behind above in front of			
understands time concepts yesterday tomorrow tomorrow night			
understands opposites bottom top go stop low high off on inside outside closed open			
can recite alphabet by rote			

COGNITIVE

Developmental Milestones	Date Achieved	NOT YET	PROGRESSING
can count to ten by rote			

understands time concepts
  on the clock
  big hand
  little hand
  when to sleep
  when school			

can trace letters			
can color within lines			
can copy shapes			

Four

Teaching Language Throughout The Day

Our emphasis in this book is on teaching specific language by using specific toys. There are many other toys that you can use as successfully as the ones we picked. There also are many other ways for you to teach language to your child. Basically, if you are paying

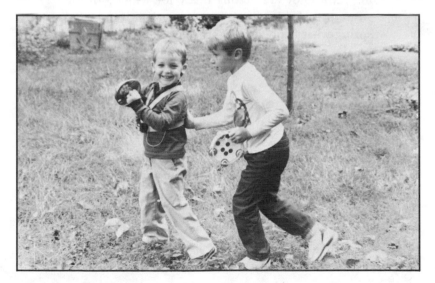

attention to your child when you are with her, you will be teaching all of the time. A beautiful way for her to learn is for you to simply talk to her in short, understandable phrases about things that she is interested in. You can discuss what you are doing, try to imagine what Grandma is doing, or show her the variety of colors in the world around her. Anything will work for you if you go about it correctly.

Going On Outings

Going for a walk on a beautiful day can be an incredible language learning time if you are willing to walk at the pace your child walks and stop for the things she wants to explore. A caterpillar crawling on the ground, a fallen leaf, a crack in the sidewalk are all new and fascinating for her. Take your time; stroll along and let her explore and ask questions about all of these wonders that she sees.

> ...Look at that beautiful red leaf. Can you find which tree it fell from? I think you're right. I think it fell from that maple tree over there. Look at all the red leaves on that maple tree. Soon they will all fall to the ground. In the summer those leaves are green. But now that it is fall, the leaves are turning red. They are getting ready for winter. In the winter all the leaves fall to the ground and next spring what happens? Right, they will all bud again on the trees....

A trip to the grocery store can be a wonderful language learning time. A little planning ahead of time can make it a learning experience for your child. Have her participate with you in the kitchen before you go to the store. The two of you look through the pantry and the refrigerator to decide what you need to buy. As you stand in front of the refrigerator, ask her if you need to get more milk. Look at the milk container and determine if it is full, empty, or almost empty. Whenever you can, give her a list that she can shop for. Use the ads in the paper to clip out pictures of items and paste them on index cards. When you make your list, choose the cards that you'll need and give them to her for her list. Since many items are the same from week to week, you can re-use your index cards each week. She may be so busy looking for her list on each aisle that you will not run into the problem of screaming for candy. If she is big enough to be out of the cart and walking around, let her take the items off the shelf herself and put them in the cart.

> ...Can you help me find the pictures of things in the paper that we need to get at the store? Let's look at this page. We need milk. Good. Let's cut out that picture and paste it on an index card. Now we also need some apples. Do you see any apples on this page? That's right, those are apples. Let's cut that out and put it on a card. What color apples do you want to get at the store? Should we get red ones or green ones? I like green ones too. We'll look for green ones when we get to the store. What else do you see that we should get?...

Continue in this way until she has a group of cards of items that she can look for when you get to the store.

Another learning opportunity is visiting friends. This often starts out as a good idea and quickly changes into a scene of screaming and fighting because your child is not properly prepared for a new environment. Planning ahead can eliminate this as well as provide an opportunity for language learning. We suggest that you have a calendar that is for your child's activities. Let's say that you are going to visit Barry and his family today. Take your child to the calendar, help her find the correct day, then take Barry's Polaroid picture (that you took before) and put it on the day of the calendar. Talk about going to Barry's house this morning and the toys that you remember that Barry has. Suggest that your child take one of her toys that Barry may not have so that they can *share* their toys. If the worst does happen and no one wants to share, then your child will have her own toy and Barry can have his. Keep your visit short and geared to the attention span of your child.

...Look at the calendar. What do we have that is special for today? Right! We are going to Barry's house. Do you remember Barry? He has a lot of cars that you like to play with. What do you have that you think Barry might like to play with? Do you want to take your new dump truck? Maybe you can build a road and play with the cars and the truck. It's always fun to share your toys with your friends....

Teaching Opportunities At Home

During the course of any ordinary day, there are numerous times for pouring language into your child. Keep her near and talk to her as much as possible about your everyday activities. You may think that this sounds like a lot of trouble but when you stop and think how short a time it really is and the value of what you are doing, you will agree that it is a small price to pay. Just think of all the things you do that you can turn into learning experiences. We have given you a few examples.

Washing Dishes

...Let's wash the dishes. We need soap and water to get the dishes clean. Look at all the bubbles. Let's take the sponge and wash the dishes clean. We can even sing a song while we wash the dishes. 'This is the way we wash the dishes, wash the dishes, wash the dishes. This is the way we wash the dishes so early in the morning.'...

Cooking

While cooking, state out loud each of the steps you're taking to put together the ingredients for the recipe.

...Let's cook some rice for dinner. You love rice. That's one of your favorite foods. We need a pot

with a lid to cook the rice. Can you help me look
in the cabinet for a pot? Here's one. Now we need
to fill the pot with water, exactly up to here. That's
two cups of water....

Vacuuming

...Time to vacuum the floor. Do you want to
be my helper? We can vacuum the floors, and
surprise Grandma and Grandpa when they come to
visit. Everything will be so clean. The vacuum will
be very loud after we plug it into the wall. We can
take turns as we vacuum....

Washing The Car

...Would you like to help me wash the car? We
need to do that because the car is very dirty. It
doesn't get a bath every night like you do. What do
we need to wash the car? Right. We need a bucket of water, some soap, and a sponge. We need all
those things to wash the car. Can you help me find
the bucket? We are going to make the car look shiny
again....

There are any number of other jobs that can be turned into fun
learning experiences including:
Ironing
Cleaning the refrigerator
Making beds
Mowing the lawn
Raking the leaves
Washing the dog
Feeding the dog or cat

Enjoy the time with your children. You are their first and best
language teacher. The relationship you establish now will last a
lifetime.

Five

Toy Safety

We have mentioned safety all along as we discussed various toys in each of the age categories. Additionally we include information here that we have obtained from the U.S. Consumer Product Safety Commission in Washington, D.C. If you have further questions you can call a Toll Free Hotline 800/638–CPSC or 800/638–2772. We encourage you to call these numbers and report any dangerous conditions that you find in any toys. This office is very interested in having up-to-date information about toy safety.

We include here some of their suggestions.

When Buying Toys

Choose toys with care. Keep in mind your child's age, interests, and skill level. Look for quality design and construction in all toys for all ages.

Make sure that all directions or instructions are clear to you, and, when appropriate, to your child. Plastic wrappings on toys should be discarded at once before they become deadly playthings.

Be a label reader. Look for, and heed, age recommendations such as "Not recommended for children under three." Look for other safety labels including: "Flame retardant/ Flame resistant" on fabric products and "Washable/hygienic materials" on stuffed toys and dolls.

When Maintaining Toys

Check all toys periodically for breakage and potential hazards. A damaged or dangerous toy should be thrown away or repaired immediately.

Edges on wooden toys that might have become sharp or surfaces covered with splinters should be sanded smooth. When repainting toys and toy boxes, avoid using old paint, since it may contain lead. New paint is regulated for lead content by the Consumer Product Safety Commission. Examine all outdoor toys regularly for rust or weak parts that could become hazardous.

When Storing Toys

Teach children to put their toys safely away on shelves or in a toy chest.

Toy boxes, too, should be checked for safety. Use a toy chest that has a lid that will stay open in any position to which it is raised and will not fall on your child. For extra safety, be sure there are ventilation holes for fresh air. Watch for sharp edges that could cut and hinges that could pinch or squeeze. See that toys used outdoors are stored after play. Rain or dew can damage a variety of toys and toy parts creating hazards.

Sharp Edges

New toys intended for children under eight years of age must, by law, be free of sharp glass and metal edges. With use, however, older toys may break, exposing cutting edges.

Small Parts

Older toys can break to reveal parts small enough to be swallowed or to become lodged in your child's windpipe, ears, or nose. The law bans small parts in new toys intended for children under three. This includes removable small eyes and noses on stuffed toys and dolls and small, removable squeakers on squeeze toys.

Loud Noises

Toy caps, some noisemaking guns, and other toys can produce sounds at noise levels that can damage hearing. The law requires the following label on boxes of caps producing noise above a certain level: "Warning—Do not fire closer than one foot to the ear. Do not use indoors." Caps producing noise that can injure a child's hearing are banned.

Cords and Strings

Toys with long strings or cords may be dangerous for infants and very young children. The cords may become wrapped around an infant's neck, causing strangulation. Never hang toys with long strings, cords, loops, or ribbons in cribs or playpens where children can become entangled.

Remove crib gyms from the crib when your child can pull himself up on his hands and knees; some children have strangled when they fell across crib gyms stretched across the crib.

Sharp Points

Toys which have been broken may have dangerous points or prongs. Stuffed toys may have wires inside the toy which could cut or stab your child if exposed. A Consumer Products Safety Commission regulation prohibits sharp points in new toys and other articles intended for use by children under eight years of age.

Propelled Objects

Your child's flying toys can be turned into weapons and cause serious injuries.

Children should never be permitted to play with adult lawn darts or other hobby or sporting equipment with sharp points. Arrows or darts used by children should have soft cork tips, rubber suction cups, or other protective tips intended to prevent injury. Check to be sure the tips are secure. Avoid those dart guns or other toys which might be capable of firing articles not intended for use in the toys such as pencils or nails.

All Toys Are Not For All Children

Keep toys designed for older children out of the hands of little ones. Follow labels that give age recommendations—some toys are recommended for older children because they may be hazardous in the hands of a younger child. Teach your older children to help keep their toys away from their younger brothers and sisters.

Even balloons when uninflated or broken can choke or suffocate your child if he tries to swallow them. More children have suffocated on uninflated balloons than on any other type of toy.

Electric Toys

Electric toys that are improperly constructed, wired, or misused can shock or burn your child. Electric toys must meet mandatory requirements for maximum surface temperatures, electrical construction, and prominent warning labels. Electric toys with heating elements are recommended only for children over eight years old. Children should be taught to use electric toys properly, cautiously, and under adult supervision.

Infant Toys

Infant toys, such as rattles, squeeze toys, and teethers, should be large enough so that they cannot enter and become lodged in your infant's throat.

The Responsibility Of The Consumer Safety Products Commission

Under the Federal Hazardous Substances Act and The Consumer Product Safety Act, the Commission has set safety regulations for certain toys and other children's articles. Manufacturers must design and manufacture their products to meet these regulations so that hazardous products are not sold.

Your Responsibility

Protecting children from unsafe toys is the responsibility of everyone. Careful toy selection and proper supervision of children at play is still the best way to protect children from toy related injuries.

Alternate Toy Sources

For many parents the cost of continually buying new and stimulating toys for their children can be prohibitive. There are several low cost alternatives to buying brand new toys. We have heard of small groups of friends who swap toys for their children for short or indefinite periods of time. This, of course, instantly increases the number of toys you and your child have to work with when doing the language development dialogues. Imagine if you were to arrange to borrow or exchange a few selected toys from one friend, a few toys from a second friend, and a few more toys from yet a third friend. You would have managed to accumulate close to a dozen different toys for you and your child to play with.

On a similar, but slightly larger scale, we have seen neighborhood groups of parents organize a toy-sharing cooperative. This can be organized on its own or as part of an already existing neighborhood organization or a community play group. Each child brings in a different toy to exchange with another child for a period of a week or two. This way, the novelty of getting a new toy never quite has time to wear off. One new toy is continually replaced by another new toy. A child's dream come true! Again, the cost of buying new toys is drastically reduced and the parents have an opportunity to see which toys their child enjoys the most before purchasing them.

Now that you have the idea of this type of alternative to buying brand-new toys in the department stores, you can see why some neighborhood preschools, special education programs, and local libraries provide this service or take it even one step further. Either for free or for a very small rental fee, you and your child can choose to borrow a toy for a designated period of time. Next time you go to your local library, find out if they have such a service. You may be surprised to find a toy lending library already in your area. Another source may be your local Association of Retarded Citizens, Easter Seals, or other special needs organizations.

Be on the lookout for garage sales and consignment shops in your area. These are two other good places to locate children's toys, often for greatly reduced prices. In these cases, the toys are often out of their boxes which gives you a chance to look them over thoroughly. You can see how interested in the toy your child is before you actually buy it.

As with all borrowed or secondhand toys, we recommend that you take special safety precautions before letting your child play with it. Wash the toys thoroughly with soap and water. Run your hand over the toy, looking for sharp or broken edges. Make sure there are no small parts that may present a danger to your child.

Toy Manufacturers

Chicco
Artsana of America, Inc.
Room 910/12, 200 5th Ave.
New York, NY 10010

Child Guidance
CBS Toys Division
500-T Harmon Meadow Blvd.
Secaucus, NJ 07094
> *Busy Bath**
> > *Registered trademark of Child Guidance.

Child Life Play Specialities, Inc.
55 Whitney Street
Holliston, MA 01746

Childcraft Education Corporation
20 Kilmer Rd.
Edison, NJ 08815

Coleco
999 Quaker Lane South
West Hartford, CT 06110
> *Scribble Stix**
> > *Registered trademark of Coleco.

Colorforms
Lash Distributors
Rochelle Park, NJ 07662
> *Wet Pets**
> *Soapy Sails Bath Toy**
> *Unimax Zoo**
> > *Registered trademarks of Lash Distributors.

Creative Aerosol Corporation
Freehold, NJ 07728
>*Funny Color Foam**
>>*Registered trademark of Creative Aerosol Corporation.

Creative Playthings, Trademark
of CBS Toys
41 Madison Ave.
New York, NY 10001

Discovery Toys
400 Ellinwood Way, Ste. 300
Pleasant Hill, CA 94523

Dolly Toy Company
Tipp City, OH 45371
>*Sesame Street Sof-Pla Blocks**
>>*Registered trademark of the Dolly Toy Company.

Eden Toys, Inc.
112 West 34th Street
New York, NY 10001

Fisher-Price Toys
East Aurora, NY 14052
>*Little People* Farm*
>*Little People* Garage*
>*Little People* Airport*
>*Little People* House*
>*Dancing Animal Music Box Mobile**
>*Play Gym*
>*Play Desk*
>*Scrub 'N Fun Center**
>*Toddler Kitchen*
>*Floating Family Water Toy*
>*Telephone Walkie Talkie*
>>*Registered trademarks of Fisher-Price.

Golden Books
Western Publishing Co., Inc.
1220 Mound Ave.
Racine, WI 53404
   *Hi-Ho Cherry-O**
      *Registered trademark of Golden Books.

Hancock Associates
Hancock, NH 03449

Horseman Dolls, Inc.
200 Fifth Avenue
New York, NY 10010

Ideal Toys
184-10 Jamaica Ave.
Hollis, NY 11423

Illco Toy Corp., Inc.
200 5th Ave.
New York, NY 10010
   Walt Disney's Mickey Mouse
   *Wash and Play Grooming Center**
      *Registered trademark of Illco Toy Corp., Inc.

James Galt & Co., Ltd.
Cheadle, Cheshire
England

Johnson and Johnson Baby
Products Co.
Grandview Rd.
Skillman, NJ 08558

Kenner Toys
1014 Vine Street
Cincinnati, OH 45202

Lego Systems, Inc.
555 Taylor Rd.
Enfield, CT 06802
*Lego Blocks**
*Registered trademark of Lego Systems, Inc.

Marx Toys, Lewish Marx and Co., Inc.
633 Hope Street
Stamford, CT 06904

Mattel, Inc.
5150 Rosecrans Ave.
Hawthorne, CA 90250
See 'N Say Zoo*
See 'N Say for Safety*
See 'N Say The Farmer Says*
*Registered trademark of Mattel.

Milton Bradley Co.
1500 Main Street
Springfield, MA 01101
*Candyland**
*Sesame Street Games for Growing**
*Registered trademarks of Milton Bradley.

Ohio Art Products
East High Street
Bryan, OH 43506

Panosh Place Learning Curves
Mt. Laurel, NJ 08054
*Curiosity Ball**
*Registered trademark of Panosh Place
Learning Curves.

Parker Brothers, Inc.
50 Dunham Rd.
Beverly, MA 01915
*Nerf Ball**
*Registered trademark of Parker Brothers.

Playskool, Inc.
1027 Newport Ave.
Pawtucket, RI 02861
>*Block Wagon**
>*Busy Box**
>*Busy Poppin' Pals**
>*Wind Up Seaplane**
>*Touch-'Ems**
>*Registered trademarks of Playskool.

Selchow & Righter Co.
2215 Union Blvd.
Bay Shore, NY 11706
>*Scrabble Alphabet Game**
>*Registered trademark of Selchow & Righter.

Sesame Street Toys and Games
International Games, Inc.
Joliet, IL 60435

Schaper Manufacturing Co.
P.O. Box 1426
Minneapolis, MN 55440

Steiff Animals
1107 Broadway
New York, NY 10010

Tonka Toys Division
Tonka Corporation
9050-T Viscount Blvd.
El Paso, TX 79925

Toys To Grow On
P.O. Box 17
Long Beach, CA 90801

Tupperware Corporation
Consumer Relations
P.O. Box 2353
Orlando, FL 32802

Walter Drake and Sons
67 Drake Building
Colorado Springs, CO 80904

Materials List

Homemade Toys

Arts And Crafts Necessities—tape, paper clips, string, paper fasteners, pipe cleaners, wire, rope, string, staples, paste, glue, tempera paint, crayons, markers, scissors, paper in various sizes and colors, stickers, paper towels, etc.

Barrels—fruit and vegetable crates.

Baskets

Boxes—all types; match boxes, gift boxes, jewelry boxes, candy boxes, etc.

Cardboard Tubing—paper towel tubing, toilet paper rolls, tin foil and plastic wrap tubing, etc.

Food Items—macaroni noodles, kidney beans, dried peas, cereal bits, etc.

Kitchen Utensils—pots, pans, measuring utensils, sifters, bowls, cooking pans, wooden spoons, spatulas, etc.

Miscellaneous Items—rubber bands, popsicle sticks, sponges, clothespins, cotton balls, cork, leaves, pine cones, small stones and shells, straws, pipe cleaners, etc.

Paper And Cardboard Items—tin foil, waxed paper, wallpaper scraps, contact paper scraps, newspaper, shirt cardboards, vegetable cartons and trays, oatmeal containers, old magazines, greeting cards, gift wrapping paper, etc.

Plastic Bottles—milk bottles, bleach bottles, dish soap dispensers, hand lotion dispensers, ketchup bottles, etc.

Plastic Containers—egg cartons, ice cream cartons, butter containers, cheese containers, egg-shaped cartons holding women's stockings, microwave dinners, etc.

Sewing Notions—yarn, decorative tape, buttons, zippers, beads, ribbons, thread, empty spools, cloth in different colors and textures, clasps, belt buckles, etc.

Styrofoam—styrofoam packing, meat trays, etc.

Places To Find Materials

Carpet Stores—carpet samples and scraps.

Fabric Stores—sewing notions, excess remnants, patches.

Garage Sales—an infinite variety of objects.

Grocery Stores—boxes, plastic and cardboard cartons, food items.

Lumber Yards—wood scraps, cinder blocks, etc.

Newspaper Companies—newsprint end-of-rolls and scraps.

Paint Stores—paint color cards.

Paper Companies—paper samples, damaged sheets of paper.

Produce Markets—vegetable and fruit crates, barrels.

Tile Companies—scraps of mosaic, ceramic, or vinyl tile.

Wallpaper Stores—out-of-date sample books, swatches.

Dramatic Play

Baskets, Grocery Carts, Bags—to go "shopping."

Boxes—to represent the stove, refrigerator, a spaceship, playhouse, etc.

Broom, Dustpan—to play clean up.

Dolls, Stuffed Animals, Furniture, And Accessories—old moving boxes for rooms, crates for beds, etc.

Empty Food Storage Cans And Boxes–to be part of the pretend kitchen.

Hats, Hats, And More Hats. Kids love them.

Miscellaneous–glasses, aprons, pocketbooks, wallets, mittens, etc.

Old Clothes–dresses, skirts, blouses, pants, slips, hats, coats, scarves, gloves. Discarded nylon nightgowns make great formal wear for kids.

Old Jewelry–bracelets, belts, necklaces, earrings, etc.

Play Money, Boxes–to play cashier.

Pots, Pans, Dishes, Cups, Eating Utensils, Paper Plates And Cups–for restaurant play, Mommy and Daddy, etc.

Telephones–a great way to practice language!

White Coats Or Shirts–to pretend to be a doctor, dentist, etc.

Resource Guide

General

American Cleft Palate Association
Nancy C. Smythe
Executive Director
1218 Grandview Ave.
University of Pittsburgh
Pittsburgh, PA 15211
412/481-1376

Academy of Aphasia
c/o Dr. Howard Gardner
Boston V.A.
Medical Center 116B
150 S. Huntington Ave.
Boston, MA 02130
617/495-4342

Association of Birth Defect
Children
Betty Mekdeci,
Executive Director
3526 Emerywood Lane
Orlando, FL 32806
305/859-2821

Association for Persons
With Severe Handicaps
Liz Lindley,
Executive Director
7010 Roosevelt Way, N.E.
Seattle, WA 98115
206/523-8446

Council for Exceptional Children
Neptha V. Greer,
Executive Director
1920 Association Dr.
Reston, VA 22091
703/620-3660

Epilepsy Foundation
of America
William McLin,
Executive Vice President
4351 Garden City Dr.
Landover, MD 20785
301/459-3700

Information Center for
Individuals With Disabilities
Lee Rachel Segal,
Executive Officer
20 Park Plaza, Room 330
617/727-5540

National Association for the
Craniofacially Handicapped
Dr. Phyllis S. Casavant,
Executive Director
P.O. Box 11082
Chattanooga, TN 37401
615/266-1632

National Center for Stuttering
Lorraine Schneider, Director
200 E. 33rd St.
New York, NY 10016
212/532-1460

National Information Center
for Handicapped Children
and Youth
Delores John, Director
P.O. Box 1492
Washington, DC 20013
703/522-3332

National Multiple
Sclerosis Society
Thor Hansen, President
205 E. 42nd St.
New York, NY 10017
212/986-3240

Autism Society of America
R. Wayne Gilpin, President
1234 Massachusetts Ave. NW
Suite 1017
Washington, DC 20005
202/783-0125

Muscular Dystrophy Association
Robert Ross, Executive Director
81 Seventh Ave.
New York, NY 10019
212/586-0808

Orton Dyslexia Society
Anne O'Flanagan,
Executive Director
724 York Rd.
Baltimore, MD 21204
301/296-0232

United Cerebral Palsy
Associations
Allin Proudfoot,
Executive Director
66 East 34th St.
New York, NY 10016
212/481-6300

Physically Handicapped

Congress of Organizations of the
Physically Handicapped
Rose Wilson, Editor
16630 Beverly
Tinley Park, IL 60477

Division for Physically
Handicapped
c/o Council for Exceptional
Children
Susan Herre, Manager
1920 Association Dr.
Reston, VA 22091
703/620-3660

National Association of the Physically Handicapped
Helen Lee Roudebush,
Administrative Assistant
76 Elm St.
London, OH 43140
614/852-1664

Learning Disabled

Association for Children and
Adults With Learning Disabilities
Jean Peterson, Executive Director
4156 Library Rd.
Pittsburgh, PA 15234
412/341-1515

Council for Learning
Disabilities
Kirsten McBridge,
Executive Director
P.O. Box 40303
Overland Park, KS 66204
913/492-3840

Foundation for Children with
Learning Disabilities
Aryln Gardner, Executive
Director
99 Park Ave. 6th Fl.
New York, NY 10016
212/687–7211

Speech And Language Disabilities

American Speech-Hearing
Association
Frederick T. Spahr, Executive
Director
10801 Rockville Pike
Rockville, MD 20852
301/897–5700

National Association for
Hearing and Speech Action
Russell L. Malone,
Executive Director
10801 Rockville Pike
Rockville, MD 20852
301/897–8682

Down Syndrome
Down's Syndrome International
Jessica M. Bennett, Administrator
11 N. 73rd Terrace, Room K
Kansas City, KN 66111
913/299–0815

National Association for
Down Syndrome
Sheila Hebein,
Executive Director
P.O. Box 4542
Oak Brook, IL 60421
312/325–9112

National Down Syndrome
Congress
Diane M. Crutcher, Executive
Director
1800 Dempster St.
Park Ridge, IL 60068
312/823–7550

National Down Syndrome
Society
Donna M. Rosenthal,
Executive Director
141 Fifth Ave.
New York, NY 10010
212/460–9330

Parents of Down's Syndrome
Children
c/o Montgomery County
Association for Retarded Citizens
11600 Nebel St.
Rockville, MD 20852
301/984-5792

Mentally Retarded

Association for Children with
Retarded Mental Development
Ida Rappaport,
Executive Director
162 Fifth Ave., 11th Fl.
New York, NY 10010
212/741-0100

Division on Mental Retardation
Council for Exceptional Children
John W. Kidd,
Executive Secretary
2372 East Broadmoor
Springfield, MO 65804
417/882-5948

Mental Retardation Association
of America
Dr. Ernest H. Dean, President
211 E. 300 South St.
Suite 212
Salt Lake City, UT 84111
801/328-1575

Association for Retarded
Citizens
Alan Abeson, Executive
Director
P.O.Box 6109
Arlington, TX 76005
817/640-0204

Division on Mental
Retardation
c/o Foundation for
Exceptional Children
Robert L. Silber, Executive
Director
1920 Association Dr.
Reston, VA 22091
703/620-3660

Retarded Infants Services
Joan M. Joseph,
Executive Director
386 Park Ave. S.
New York, NY 10016
212/889-5464

Visually Handicapped

American Council of the
Blind Parents
c/o American Council of the Blind
Roy J. Ward, President
1010 Vermont Ave., NW
Suite 1100
Washington, DC 20005
804/288-0395

American Foundation
for the Blind
William F. Gallagher, Executive
Director
15 West 16th St.
New York, NY 10011
212/620-2000

International Institute for
Visually Impaired
Sherry Raynor, President
1975 Rutgers Circle
East Lansing, MI 48823
517/332-2666

Association for the
Education of the Visually
Handicapped
Kathleen Megivern,
Executive Director
206 N. Washington St.
Suite 320
Alexandria, VA 22314
703/548-1884

Division for the Visually
Handicapped
c/o Council for Exceptional
Children
Vincent M. McVeigh,
President
1920 Association Dr.
Reston, VA 22091

National Association for
Visually Handicapped
Lorraine Marchi,
Executive Director
22 W. 21st St.
New York, NY 10010
212/889-3141

Blind-Retarded

Association for Advancement of
Blind and Retarded
Max Posner, Executive Director
16409 Hillside Ave.
Jamaica, NY 11432
718/523-2222

Deaf-Blind

American Association for
Deaf-Blind
Rod Madonald, President
814 Thayer Ave.
Silver Spring, MD 20910
301/588-6545

Helen Keller National
Center for Deaf-Blind
Youths and Adults
Martin A. Adler, Director
111 Middle Neck Rd.
Sands Point, NY 11050
516/944-8900

Hearing Impaired

Alexander Graham Bell
Association for the Deaf
Donna McCord Dickman,
Executive Director
3417 Volta Pl., NW
Washington, DC 20007
202/337-5220

American Society for Deaf
Children
Millie Maisel,
Administrative Assistant
814 Thayer Ave.
Silver Spring, MD 20901
301/585-5400

National Association of the Deaf
Gary Olsen, Executive Director
814 Thayer Ave.
Silver Spring, MD 20901
301/587-1788

International Organization
for the Education of the
Hearing Impaired
Sandy North, Chairperson
3417 Volta Pl., NW
Washington, DC 20007
202/337-5220

International Parents'
Organization
c/o Alexander Graham Bell
Association for the Deaf
Bruce Goldstein, Chairperson
1537 35th St. NW
Washington, DC 20007
202/337-5220

National Center for Law
and the Deaf
Sy DuBow, Legal Director
800 Florida Ave, NE
Washington, DC 20002
202/651-5373

National Foundation for
Children's Hearing Education and
Research
928 McLean Ave.
Yonkers, NY 10704
914/237-2676

Council on Education of the
Deaf
Dr. Don Hicks, Executive
Director
800 Florida Ave., NE
Washington, DC 20002
202/651-5020

National Cued Speech
Association
Mary Elsie Sbaiti, President
P.O. Box 31345
Raleigh, NC 27622
919/828-1218

Self-Help for Hard of
Hearing People
Howard E. Stone, Founder
7800 Wisconsin Ave.
Bethesda, MD 20814
301/657-2248

Sources For Information About Children's Books

Children's Book Council, Inc.
67 Irving Place
New York, NY 10003

Children's Books in Print
(revised annually)
R. R. Bowker
245 West 17th St.
New York, NY 10011

Sesame Street Magazine
P.O. Box 2896
Boulder, CO 80321

Horn Book Magazine
Park Square Building
31 St. James Avenue
Boston, MA 02116

A Parent's Guide to
Children's Reading
by Nancy Larrick
Bantam Books
New York, NY

Highlights for Children
2300 West Fifth Ave.
P.O. Box 269
Columbus, OH 43216-0269

References

Almy, Millie and Cunningham, Ruth. *Ways of Studying Children*, New York: Teachers College, Columbia University: Teachers College Press, 1959.

Atack, M. Sally. *Art Activities for the Handicapped*, Englewood Cliffs, NJ: Prentice-Hall, Inc., 1986.

Bangs, Tina. *Birth To Three — Developmental Learning And The Handicapped Child*, Teaching Resources Corporation, 50 Pond Park Road, Hingham, MA 02043: A New York Times Co., 1979.

Barber, W. Lucie and Williams, Herman. *Your Baby's First 30 Months*, H.P. Books, P.O. Box 5367, Tucson, AZ 85703: Fisher Publishing Co., 1981.

Breger, Louis. *From Instinct To Identity — The Development Of Personality*, Englewood Cliffs, NJ: Prentice-Hall, Inc., 1974.

Brazelton, T. Berry. *Infants and Mothers*, New York: Dell Publishing Co., 1969.

Burtt, Kent Garland and Kalkstein, Karen. *Smart Toys: For Babies From Birth To Two*, New York: Harper and Row, Publishers, Inc., 1981.

Caplan, Frank and Theresa. *The Power of Play*, Garden City, NY: Anchor Press/Doubleday, 1973.

Carney, Steven. *Toy Book*, New York: Workman Publishing Co., 1972.

Einon, Dorothy. *Play With A Purpose: Learning Games For Children 6 Weeks To 2-3 Year Olds*, New York: St. Martin's Press, 1985.

Eliason, F. Claudie and Jenkins, Lea Thomson. *A Preschool Guide To Early Childhood Curriculum*, St. Louis: The C.V. Mosby Co., 1977.

Engel, C. Rose. *Language Motivating Experiences For Young Children: Educative Toys and Supplies*, Van Nuys, CA, 1968.

Erickson, H. Erik. *Childhood And Society*, New York: W.W. Norton & Co., 1963.

Garvey, Catharine. *Children's Talk*, Boston: Harvard University Press, 1984.

Goldberg, Sally. *Teaching With Toys,* Ann Arbor: The University of Michigan Press, 1981.

Gordon, J. Ira. *Baby Learning Through Baby Play,* New York: St. Martin's Press, 1970.

Gordon, J. Ira; Guinah, Barry; Jestes, R. Emile. *The Instruction for the Development of Human Resources,* Gainesville: University of Florida.

Gordon, J. Ira. *Baby to Parent, Parent to Baby,* New York: St. Martin's Press, 1977.

Gordon, J. Ira. *Child Learning Through Child Play: Learning Activities for 2-3 Year Olds,* New York: St. Martin's Press, 1972.

Hagstrom, Julie and Morrill, Joan. *Games Babies Play and More Games Babies Play,* New York: Pocket Books, 1981.

Hendrick, Joanne. *The Whole Child, New Trends In Early Education,* St. Louis: The C.V. Mosby Co., 1975.

Hogan, James Lorene (Sister). *The What, When And How Of Teaching Language To Deaf Children (for preschool and primary grades),* Wydown and Big Berd Boulevards, St. Louis, MO: CSJ Forthborne College, 1968.

Houghton, Janaye Matteson. *Homespun Language,* Whitehaven Publishing Co., Inc., 1982.

Ilg, L. Frances, M.D.; Ames, Louis Bates, Ph.D.; Beeker, Sidney M., M.D. *Child Behavior,* New York: Harper and Row, Publishers, 1981.

Isaacs, Susan. *Intellectual Growth In Young Children,* New York: Schocken Books, 1972.

Johnson, Doris McNeely. *The Creative Parenting Toy Guide,* self-published, 1980.

Kaban, Barbara. Foreword by White, Burton L. *Choosing Toys For Children From Birth To Five,* New York: Schocken Books, 1979.

Karnes, B. Merle. *You And Your Small Wonder, Book 2:18-36 Months,* Circle Pines, MN 55014: American Guidance Service, 1982.

LaCross, R.F.; Litman, F.; Oglivie, D.M.; White, B.L. *The Preschool Project: Experience and the Development of Human Competence in the First Six Years of Life,* Monograph No. 9, Boston: Harvard University Publications Office, 1969.

Markun, Patricia Maloney. *Play: Children's Business,* 3615 Wisconsin Ave. NW, Washington, D.C.: Association for Childhood Education International, 1974.

Maryland State Department of Education. *Parent Helper, Handicapped Children Birth to Five—Communication*, Division of Special Education, 1982.

Marzollo, Jean and Harper, Janice Lloyd. *Learning Through Play*, New York: Harper and Row, Publishers, 1972.

Mattersoh, E.M. *Play And Playthings For The Preschool Child*, Baltimore, MD: Penguin Books, 1967.

McConley, Roy and Jeffree, Dorothy. *Making Toys For Handicapped Children*, Englewood Cliffs, NJ 07632: Prentice-Hall.

Millnard, Joan and Behrmann, Polly. *Parents As Playmates—A Games Approach To The Preschool Years*, New York: Human Sciences Press, 1979.

Monsees, K. Edna. *Structured Language For Children With Special Language Learning Problems*, Children's Hospital of the District of Columbia, Washington, D.C. 20001: Children's Hearing and Speech Center, 1972.

Munger, Evelyn Moats and Bowdon, Susan Jane. *Child Play Activities For Your Child's First Three Years*, New York: E.P. Dutton, Inc., 1983.

O'Neill, Mary. *Hailstones and Halibut Bones*, Doubleday and Co., 1961.

Oppenheim, Joanne F. *Kids And Play*, New York: Ballantine Books, 1984.

Powers, Margaret Hall, "Functional Disorders of Articulation/Symptomotology and Etiology." In *Handbook of Speech Pathology and Andiology*, edited by Lee Edward Travis, 842. Englewood Cliffs: Prentice Hall, 1971.

Pushaw, David. *Teach Your Child To Talk*, New York: CEBCO Standard Publishing, 1976.

Schwartz, Sue (Ed.) *Choices In Deafness: A Parents Guide*, Kensington, MD: Woodbine House, 1987.

Sternlicht, Nanny, Ph.D. *Games Children Play*, Abraham Hurwitz Yeshiva University Staten Island, Developmental Center, New York: Reinhold Co., 1981.

Spock, Benjamin. *The Best Toys For Kids (and the Worst)*. Redbook, November 1985, pp. 16, 18.

Stray-Gundersen, Karen (Ed.) *Babies With Down Syndrome: A New Parents Guide*, Kensington, MD: Woodbine House, 1986.

Van Riper, Charles. *Teaching Your Child to Talk*, New York: Harper & Row, 1960.

Wholley, L. Donald and Malott, W. Richard. *Elementary Principles of Behavior*, Englewood Cliffs, NJ: Prentice-Hall, Inc., 1970.

Index

About The Authors

Sue Schwartz, Ph.D.

Sue Schwartz received her Master's degree in Speech and Hearing from Central Institute for the Deaf in St. Louis, Missouri and her Ph.D. in Curriculum and Instruction with an emphasis in Family Counseling from the University of Maryland.

Dr. Schwartz developed the Parent Infant Auditory Program in the Montgomery County Public Schools. In this capacity she has worked with parents and recognized the need for parents to have a clear understanding of how to teach language skills to children with special needs.

She is the editor of *Choices In Deafness: A Parents Guide*. (Woodbine House, 1987).

Joan E. Heller Miller, Ed.M.

Joan Miller received her Master's degree in Education from Harvard University with an emphasis in Counseling and Consulting Psychology. She did her undergraduate training at Tufts University in early childhood education and mental health. She is a certified teacher in early childhood education, and has worked extensively teaching and counseling special needs children and their families. Joan teaches a college course on Deafness and Communication and is the parent of a hearing impaired daughter.